Congenital Hand Differences

Guest Editor

KEVIN C. CHUNG, MD

HAND CLINICS

www.hand.theclinics.com

May 2009 • Volume 25 • Number 2

SAUNDERS an imprint of ELSEVIER, Inc.

W.B. SAUNDERS COMPANY
A Division of Elsevier Inc.

1600 John F. Kennedy Blvd. ● Suite 1800 ● Philadelphia, Pennsylvania 19103

http://www.theclinics.com

HAND CLINICS Volume 25, Number 2
May 2009 ISSN 0749-0712, ISBN-13: 978-1-4377-0483-9, ISBN-10: 1-4377-0483-2

Editor: Debora Dellapena

Hand Clinics (ISSN 0749-0712) is published quarterly by Elsevier Inc., 360 Park Avenue South, New York, NY 10010-1710. Months of publication are February, May, August, and November. Business and Editorial Offices: 1600 John F. Kennedy Blvd., Suite 1800, Philadelphia, PA 19103-2899. Customer Service Office: 11830 Westline Industrial Drive, St. Louis, MO 63146. Periodicals postage paid at New York, NY, and additional mailing offices. Subscription price is $282.00 per year (domestic individuals), $446.00 per year (domestic institutions), $144.00 per year (domestic students/residents), $321.00 per year (Canadian individuals), $510.00 per year (Canadian institutions), $383.00 per year (international individuals), $510.00 per year (international institutions), and $189.00 per year (international and Canadian students/residents). Foreign air speed delivery is included in all *Clinics* subscription prices. All prices are subject to change without notice. **POSTMASTER:** Send address changes to *Hand Clinics*, 11830 Westline Industrial Drive, St. Louis, MO 63146. Customer Service (orders, claims, online, change of address): Elsevier Periodicals Customer Service, 11830 Westline Industrial Drive, St. Louis, MO 63146. Tel: 1-800-654-2452 (U.S. and Canada). Fax: 314-523-5170. E-mail: journalscustomerservice-usa@elsevier.com (for print support); journalsonlinesupport-usa@elsevier.com (for online support).

Reprints. For copies of 100 or more of articles in this publication, please contact the Commercial Reprints Department, Elsevier Inc., 360 Park Avenue South, New York, New York 10010-1710. Tel.: 212-633-3812; Fax: 212-462-1935; E-mail: reprints@elsevier.com.

Hand Clinics is covered in *MEDLINE/PubMed (Index Medicus)*, *Current Contents/Clinical Medicine*, *EMBASE/Excerpta Medica*, and *ISI/BIOMED*.

Printed and bound in the United Kingdom

Transferred to Digital Print 2011

Contributors

GUEST EDITOR

KEVIN C. CHUNG, MD
Professor of Surgery, Section of Plastic
Surgery, Department of Surgery; and Assistant
Dean for Faculty Affairs (Instructional Track),
The University of Michigan Medical School,
Ann Arbor, Michigan

AUTHORS

MATTHEW J. CARTY, MD
Fellow, Hand and Microsurgery, Beth Israel
Deaconess Medical Center, Harvard Medical
School, Boston, Massachusetts

KEVIN C. CHUNG, MD
Professor of Surgery, Section of Plastic
Surgery, Department of Surgery; and Assistant
Dean for Faculty Affairs (Instructional Track),
The University of Michigan Medical School,
Ann Arbor, Michigan

CHARLES A. GOLDFARB, MD
Associate Professor, Department of
Orthopaedic Surgery, Washington University
School of Medicine at Barnes Jewish Hospital,
St. Louis, Missouri

MICHELLE A. JAMES, MD
Chief, Department of Orthopaedic Surgery,
Shriners Hospital for Children Northern
California; Professor, Department of
Orthopaedic Surgery; and Chief, Division of
Pediatric Orthopaedics, University of California
Davis School of Medicine, Sacramento,
California

NEIL F. JONES, MD
Professor and Chief of Hand Surgery,
Department of Orthopedic Surgery, Division of
Plastic and Reconstructive Surgery, University
of California-Irvine Medical Center, Orange,
California

KENJI KAWAMURA, MD, PhD
Assistant Professor, Department of
Orthopaedic Surgery, Nara Medical University,
Kashihara, Nara, Japan

SCOTT H. KOZIN, MD
Clinical Professor, Department of Orthopaedic
Surgery, Temple University; Director, Upper
Extremity Center of Excellence, Shriners
Hospitals for Children, Philadelphia,
Pennsylvania

PAUL R. MANSKE, MD
Professor of Orthopedic Surgery, Department
of Orthopaedic Surgery, Washington University
School of Medicine, St. Louis, Missouri

MICHAEL L. NGUYEN, MD
Department of Orthopedic Surgery, University
of California-Irvine Medical Center, Orange,
California

DOUGLAS M. SAMMER, MD
Assistant Professor, Division of Plastic
Surgery, Department of Surgery, Washington
University, St. Louis, Missouri

AMIR TAGHINIA, MD
Instructor, Department of Surgery, Children's
Hospital Boston; Instructor, Department of
Surgery, Beth Israel Deaconess Medical
Center, Harvard Medical School, Boston,
Massachusetts

MICHAEL A. TONKIN, MBBS, MD, FRACS, FRCS EdOrth
Professor, Department of Hand Surgery and Peripheral Nerve Surgery, Royal North Shore Hospital, University of Sydney, Sydney, Australia

JENNIFER M. TY, MD
Director, Hand and Upper Extremity Division, Department of Orthopaedic Surgery, Alfred I. duPont Hospital for Children, Nemours, Wilmington, Delaware

JOSEPH UPTON, MD
Associate Professor, Department of Surgery, Children's Hospital Boston; Associate Professor, Shriners Hospital Boston, Harvard Medical School, Boston, Massachusetts

ANDREW J. WATT, MD
Division of Plastic and Reconstructive Surgery, Department of Surgery, Stanford University Hospitals and Clinics, Palo Alto, California

Contents

Congenital Hand Differences: Embryology and Classification

Douglas M. Sammer and Kevin C. Chung

> Congenital hand differences affect approximately 1 in 500 persons and present unique diagnostic and classification challenges. The embryology of the hand and upper extremity is discussed, including the molecular basis for patterning of the upper limb. The Swanson/International Federation of Societies for Surgery of the Hand classification system is described, along with a discussion of the difficulties in classifying congenital hand differences based on morphology or etiology.

Congenital Failure of Formation of the Upper Limb

Paul R. Manske and Charles A. Goldfarb

> This article provides an overview of the various classification systems for radial longitudinal, central longitudinal, and ulnar longitudinal deficiencies. It looks specifically at radius deficiency, hypoplastic thumb, index finger pollicization, narrowed thumb web, forearm-elbow deformities, and hand abnormalities. Various surgical approaches to these conditions and their results are explored. The authors conclude that longitudinal failure of formation deformities comprises a substantial portion of the anomalies of the upper limb. Although much of the past and current congenital hand literature has been devoted to these conditions, they continue to be a reconstructive challenge to hand surgeons involved in their care.

Failure of Differentiation Part I: Syndactyly

Michael A. Tonkin

> Syndactyly is one of the two most common congenital hand anomalies, the other being polydactyly. Traditionally, syndactyly is considered simple when only skin is involved; complex when there is bone connection; complete when the web involvement includes the nail folds; incomplete or partial when the nail folds are not involved, but when the web depth is distal to its normal position; and complicated when there are multiple tissue abnormalities. This article discusses the various types of syndactyly, the current state of known genetic mechanisms, and the author's preferred surgical techniques for correction.

Failure of Differentiation: Part II (Arthrogryposis, Camptodactyly, Clinodactyly, Madelung Deformity, Trigger Finger, and Trigger Thumb)

Jennifer M. Ty and Michelle A. James

> The term "failure of differentiation" describes the phenotypes of a large number of otherwise unrelated conditions. The six conditions described here (arthrogryposis, camptodactyly, clinodactyly, Madelung deformity, trigger finger, and trigger thumb) are believed to occur because various structures failed to differentiate normally;

however, they have neither common features nor a common cause. We have included information about the history and diagnosis of these conditions, the cause (if known), and the current concepts of treatment and expected outcomes.

Congenital limb duplications include pre- and post-axial polydactyly, central polydactyly, and the mirror-hand spectrum. Treatment of these duplications constitutes a significant functional and aesthetic challenge for the reconstructive hand surgeon. This article provides an inclusive review of the embryologic and molecular mechanisms underlying these deformities and focuses on their clinical treatment. The anatomic variation, classification, surgical treatment, and outcomes of surgical intervention are reviewed for each of the disorders of duplication.

Over the past five decades, one of the major problems in the treatment of overgrowth syndromes of the hand has been classification. Currently, a number of specific conditions with known natural histories have been delineated and reviewed. Treatment is highly individualized. Amputation is still recommended for grotesque deformities of the upper limb. Early aggressive surgery, when indicated, will improve contour, function, and appearance. Specific therapeutic techniques include radical debulking, microvascular neurolysis, vascular reconstruction, epiphysiodesis, and, in some cases, thumb or digit replacement. Long-term outcomes remain in the good-to-fair range and are dependent upon the condition, reconstructive techniques employed, age of patient, and the severity of deformity.

Brachydactyly simply means "short finger", but it has a clinical spectrum ranging from minor digital hypoplasia to complete aplasia. The index and small fingers are the most commonly affected digits, and the middle phalanx is the most commonly affected bone. Presentation of brachydactyly is highly variable—a digit may be just slightly shorter because of reduced growth of one phalanx or the metacarpal, or there may be complete absence of one or more phalanges, or there may be complete aplasia of the digit or multiple digits. This article discusses the results of conventional reconstruction using nonvascularized toe phalangeal bone grafting and distraction lengthening and the newer technique of microsurgical toe-to-hand transfers.

Constriction band syndrome is an uncommon congenital abnormality with multiple disfiguring and disabling manifestations. Early amnion rupture with subsequent entanglement of fetal parts by amniotic strands is currently the primary theory for the development of this syndrome. Management of constriction band syndrome is focused on improving function and development while providing a more acceptable esthetic appearance. The treatment should be tailored to the individual. Timing of repair and surgical planning are important to provide the best functional results for affected hands.

Generalized Skeletal Abnormalities

Andrew J. Watt and Kevin C. Chung

Given the complexity and diversity of congenital differences, a separate and broad category of generalized skeletal abnormalities was proposed to include all conditions that are unable to be neatly packaged into the other categories. Some of the conditions included in this category are obscure, whereas others are more common. Some conditions listed in this section may fit into other categories but may be considered as part of the overall classification scheme. This article presents congenital trigger finger, congenital clasped thumb, Madelung's deformity, and other skeletal hand deformities that are characteristic of generalized bone and connective tissue disorders, including achondroplasia and Marfan syndrome.

Congenital Differences About the Elbow

Scott H. Kozin

The elbow is frequently affected by congenital differences that limit flexion–extension and supination–pronation. The limitation can occur in utero or develop over time. Delayed causes usually gradually disrupt the anatomy and function of the paired bone forearm. Accurate diagnosis is based on a careful examination and perusal of radiographs. Certain diagnoses can be helped by surgery and will result in improved limb usage and function. In contrast, other diagnoses are recalcitrant to modern operative techniques but will benefit from occupational therapy and adaptive equipment to enhance independence and activities essential to daily life. This article discusses diagnosis and treatment of synostosis, arthrogryposis, pterygium, multiple hereditary exostosis, and the unsalvageable forearm.

Congenital Hand Surgery: What's New and What's Coming

Charles A. Goldfarb

Congenital hand surgery has advanced during the last 10 years with surgical technique improvements, the incorporation of new technologies, and an enhanced understanding of the basic pathology of upper extremity anomalies. This article reviews the literature with a survey of 70 articles from seven leading journals published in the last 12 years. The author concludes that the next decade should be even more exciting with the incorporation of an improved understanding of tissue engineering and molecular genetics into classification and treatment algorithms. Understanding the genetic pathways of normal, and therefore abnormal, development should allow improved classification schemes and intervention to prevent, modify, or remedy these birth abnormalities.

Index

Hand Clinics

THE CLINICS ARE NOW AVAILABLE ONLINE!

Access your subscription at:
www.theclinics.com

Preface

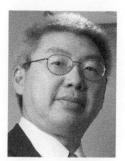

Kevin C. Chung, MD
Guest Editor

The most enticing and challenging component of a hand surgery practice is the treatment of children who have congenital hand differences. Children are incredibly adaptable, and they can compensate remarkably well, despite missing a major portion of a limb. The difficulty in treating children's hands is not only what to do and how to do it, but when to do it and when not to do it. For example, children who have syndactyl of border digits need to have earlier operations, perhaps before the age of 6 months, to avoid permanent contractures of the joints that can inevitably result in irrevocable deformities. Similarly, newborns who have constriction band syndrome may require early releases of the constriction band to preserve the length of the already short digits. In contrast, some of the more dramatic hand problems, such as cleft hands, may not require treatment, and inconsiderate operations may result in an aesthetic triumph, but a functional disaster.

The creative and caring qualities of pediatric hand surgery are fully displayed by the contributing authors in this issue. Their meticulous presentation of sage experiences in their articles share the loving relationships with the children whose future livelihood depends on the successful treatments. I am most privileged to have assembled some of the world's leading experts in treating congenital hand problems. My assignment as the editor for this issue was made simple by my dear friends, who contributed magnificent and scholarly manuscripts that required virtually no editing. The authors for this issue were selected for their experience and insights to these complex problems. Treating pediatric hand problems is not an exact science, because it is impossible to perform high-level evidence studies because of ethical concerns and the relatively low incidence of these conditions. Therefore, the expert opinions by trusted senior colleagues are all we have to go by. It is with this duty that the authors in this issue present time-tested procedures that can ensure predictably acceptable outcomes based on a logical sequence of treatments to enhance the children's potential. Certainly, this issue does not cover all the complexities of this subject, but it does synthesize a crucial element of practical approaches in treating common congenital hand problems.

I am grateful for the opportunity to have children as a large component of my practice. Many of them travel quite a distance to seek my care, and I consider them my children, as I see them transitioning from newborns to college students. We all hope that the advances in medical technology and tissue engineering will allow us to provide even more options to the children whose parents have entrusted the care of their children to us. I am indebted to Allison Pushman, my assistant (who will enter medical school next year) for her expert coordination of this project. I am proud to present this issue to you and on behalf of my contributing authors, thank you for your devotion to the children.

Kevin C. Chung, MD
Section of Plastic Surgery
Department of Surgery
University of Michigan Medical School
2130 Taubman Center
1500 E. Medical Center Drive
Ann Arbor, MI 48109, USA

E-mail address:
kecchung@umich.edu (K.C. Chung)

Hand Clin 25 (2009) ix
doi:10.1016/j.hcl.2009.02.001

Congenital Hand Differences: Embryology and Classification

Douglas M. Sammer, MD[a], Kevin C. Chung, MD[b],*

KEYWORDS

- Congenital • Hand • Classification • Embryology
- Anomaly • Malformation • Differences • Pediatric

The prevalence of upper limb congenital differences is approximately 1 in 500 persons[1] and varies within different populations and ethnic groups. The true incidence is not known, however, because other associated anomalies often result in spontaneous prenatal loss. In addition, some forms of congenital hand difference may go unrecorded (eg, mild camptodactyly), making it difficult to ascertain their prevalence.[2,3] It is known that the incidence of congenital hand differences increases with maternal age and with pre- or post-term birth.[1] It should be remembered that approximately half of those born with an upper limb congenital difference have another anomaly not associated with a hand. Most cases are attributable to inherited or spontaneous genetic alterations and are less often caused by environmental agents (teratogens).[4]

EMBRYOLOGY

The embryologic limb bud can first be seen at just less than 4 weeks after fertilization, and by 8 weeks, all upper extremity structures can be identified.[5] It is during this 4-week time frame that most congenital upper limb differences arise.[5] For 8 weeks after fertilization, the existing fetal limb structures continue to grow and develop.

Limb bud development begins with mesodermal protrusion into the enveloping ectoderm on the ventrolateral aspect of the embryo. Mesoderm originating from somites (lateral to the early spinal cord) differentiates into upper extremity skeletal muscle, and mesoderm originating from the lateral plates (ventral and lateral to the endoderm) differentiates into cartilage and bone (**Fig. 1**).[6] As the limb bud develops, chondrification of the skeleton occurs in a proximal-to-distal direction and is completed by approximately 50 days. Joint development also occurs in a proximal-to-distal direction through a process called cavitation. By 37 days, the hand plate is well developed. Digital rays arise, and finger separation is seen between 47 and 53 days.[5,7] All skeletal muscles are present by 7 weeks.[7] Ossification of the cartilaginous skeleton (endochondral ossification) begins after the fetal period commences and continues postnatally.

The subclavian artery is present by the third week, and upper extremity vasculature can be identified at 30 days after fertilization. The first branch to arise from the brachial artery is the median artery, which courses along the midline of the developing forearm. The ulnar artery develops subsequently, giving rise to the deep palmar arch in the hand. The radial artery develops last, followed by diminution of the median artery.[8]

Peripheral nerve development follows vascular development, and nerves are first seen in the extremities at approximately 36 days after

Supported in part by a Midcareer Investigator Award in Patient-Oriented Research (K24AR053120) from the National Institute of Arthritis and Musculoskeletal and Skin Diseases.

[a] Division of Plastic Surgery, Department of Surgery, Washington University, 660 South Euclic Avenue, Suite 1150, St. Louis, MO 63110, USA

[b] Section of Plastic Surgery, Department of Surgery, University of Michigan Medical School, 2130 Taubman Center, 1500 E. Medical Center Drive, Ann Arbor, MI 48109–0340, USA

* Corresponding author.

E-mail address: kecchung@umich.edu (K.C. Chung).

Hand Clin 25 (2009) 151–156
doi:10.1016/j.hcl.2009.02.002

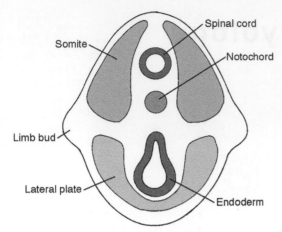

Fig. 1. Axial view of the embryo at approximately 4 weeks of gestation. Somatic mesoderm and lateral plate mesoderm contribute to the developing limb buds.

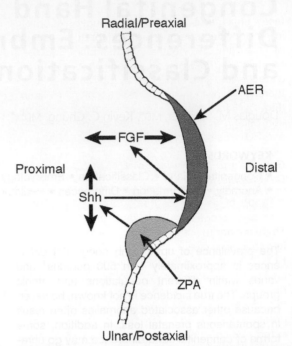

Fig. 2. AER and the zone of polarizing activity (ZPA) control the proximal-distal and radial-ulnar axes, respectively. Proximal-distal growth is controlled by FGF, and radio-ulnar differentiation is controlled by Sonic hedgehog (Shh). Shh also stimulates FGF production by the AER.

fertilization.[7] The neural tube gives rise to sensory nerves, whereas the motor nerves develop from tissue originating in the neural crest.[9] Mixed sensory and motor nerve roots form from C6 through T1, followed by sprouting axons that attach to developing muscles in the growing extremity.[9]

Three Axes of Development

Limb growth and differentiation progress along three axes: proximodistal (PD), anteroposterior (AP), and dorsoventral (DV).[6] The PD axis refers to elongation of the limb, the AP axis defines radio-ulnar or preaxial or postaxial orientation, and the DV axis provides dorsal and palmar orientation.[6] The AP axis is defined first, followed by the DV axis and the PD axis.

The PD axis is the last axis established and is controlled by the apical ectodermal ridge (AER), a thickened ridge of ectoderm that develops in the area in which the limb bud begins to grow.[6] The AER is known to secrete several fibroblast growth factors (FGFs), including FGF-2, FGF-4, and FGF-8, that provide the molecular control for the AER and for the differentiation and growth along the PD axis.[10–12] The mesoderm also plays a role in establishment of the PD axis by stimulating the AER to produce FGF (Fig. 2).[13] The role of the AER in PD development is demonstrated in experimental models in which excision of the AER causes truncation of the developing extremity, whereas implantation of the AER at another site results in development of an ectopic limb.[14]

The AP axis (preaxial or postaxial, or radioulnar axis) is the first axis to be established, and its orientation is defined before the limb bud is present. A focus of specialized mesodermal tissue in what later becomes the posterior (postaxial or ulnar) aspect of the limb begins to secrete a protein that controls differentiation and growth along the AP axis. This focus of tissue is called the zone of polarizing activity (ZPA), and the protein produced is Sonic hedgehog (Shh) (see Fig. 2).[6] The influence of the ZPA in defining the AP axis has been demonstrated in experimental models, in which transplantation of the ZPA to the preaxial (radial) side of the developing limb results in mirror duplication of the ulnar side.[14] Duplication of the ZPA has been implicated in the development of mirror hand in humans. Although Shh controls and is necessary for AP polarization and AP growth, it also plays a role in PD growth. It does this by stimulating FGF-4 production by the AER (see Fig. 2). In fact, without the stimulation provided by Shh from the ZPA, the AER is no longer effective and PD growth halts.[15,16]

The establishment and control of the DV axis are not as well understood as those of the other two axes.[6] The dorsal ectoderm produces a protein called wingless-type mouse mammary tumor virus integration site family member 7a (Wnt-7a). Wnt-7a, in turn, induces production of transcription factor Lmx1. Wnt-7a–induced production of Lmx1 in the dorsal ectoderm is required for dorsalization of the limb.[17] Another transcription factor, engrailed-1 (En-1) is produced on the ventral aspect of the limb and blocks Wnt-7a expression, thereby allowing ventralization of the limb (**Fig. 3**).[18] In addition, Wnt-7a promotes production of Shh in the ZPA, thereby affecting the AP and PD axes secondarily.[17]

Genetic and Molecular Control of Limb Development

A group of genes, the homeobox (HOX) genes, also play a critical role in limb embryogenesis. There are approximately 40 HOX genes, organized into four gene clusters (HOXA, HOXB, HOXC, and HOXD). Each of the four HOX groups is located on a separate chromosome, and each gene tends to be expressed in a different anatomic location in the nascent limb.[6] Defects in various HOX genes, particularly in the HOXD cluster, have been implicated in several common congenital hand differences.[19] At least one type of synpolydactyly is known to be caused by mutations in the HOXD13 gene,[20] and HOXD13 and HOXA13 have been implicated in the formation of monodactylous limbs and development of hand-foot-genital syndrome.[21,22]

The genetics and molecular control of congenital hand differences are extremely complex and involve interaction between a multitude of genes and proteins, whose expression and production in time and space are precisely coordinated. In addition, environmental factors interact with genetic and molecular events to alter and modify the course of limb differentiation and growth. Although tremendous progress has been made in understanding this complex interplay, these events are only beginning to be elucidated.

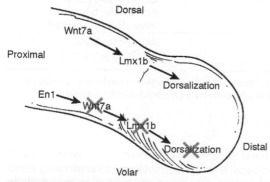

Fig. 3. Dorsal surface of the limb bud produces a protein, Wnt-7a, which causes production of transcription factor Lmx1b, leading to dorsalization. On the volar aspect, En-1 inhibits Wnt-7a, thereby blocking dorsalization and allowing ventralization.

CLASSIFICATION SYSTEMS

For many years, a wide assortment of Greek and Latin words was used to describe various congenital hand differences. Swanson and his colleagues[23,24] made the point that this amounted to nothing more than using a foreign language to describe the anomaly, which did little to classify or categorize it. An ideal classification system for congenital hand differences should incorporate etiology, diagnosis, treatment, and prognosis. It should be detailed enough to differentiate among various differences but should not be too cumbersome to be useful.[25] It should also be widely or universally accepted and used, so that standardized communication and investigation are possible. As our understanding of congenital hand differences has evolved, various classification systems have been proposed. As our understanding of the genetic and molecular bases of congenital hand differences become deeper, and as novel treatment strategies are developed, new classification systems are likely to be devised.

Swanson/International Federation of Societies for Surgery of the Hand Classification System

In 1976, the American Society for Surgery of the Hand and International Federation of Societies for Surgery of the Hand (IFSSH) adopted a classification system that was first proposed by Swanson in 1964.[26] Although it has been modified since then, the original scheme remains largely unchanged.[23,24] This system divides congenital hand differences into seven main categories that are further divided into subcategory, level of anomaly, diagnosis (nomenclature), and subclassification (**Table 1**).[23] Category I consists of "failure of formation" and is subcategorized into transverse and longitudinal arrests. Transverse arrests are further classified based on the level of arrest, whereas longitudinal arrests are divided into preaxial, postaxial, central, and intersegmental arrests. Phocomelia is an example of intersegmental longitudinal arrest, in which a segment of the extremity between the shoulder and the hand is absent.

Category II consists of "failure of differentiation" and is subcategorized into soft tissue, skeletal, and tumorous anomalies. Soft tissue and skeletal anomalies are further classified according to anatomic location, and tumorous anomalies are classified based on the type of tissue involved (ie, hemangioma, lymphatic malformation). Syndactyly and forearm synostosis are examples of failure of differentiation. Category III includes "duplication" and is subcategorized by the anatomic area affected. Polydactyly and mirror

Table 1
Abbreviated 1983 Swanson/International Federation of Societies for Surgery of the Hand classification

Main Category	Subcategory	Level	Diagnosis (Example)
I. Failure of formation (arrest)	Transverse longitudinal	Shoulder Arm Elbow Forearm Wrist Carpus Metacarpal Phalanx Radial Ulnar Central Intersegmental	Amelia Radial club Cleft hand (typical/atypical) Phocomelia
II. Failure of differentiation (separation)	Soft tissue Skeletal Tumorous	Disseminated Shoulder Elbow and forearm Wrist and hand Shoulder Elbow Forearm Wrist and hand "Hemangiotic" Lymphatic Neurogenic Connective tissue Skeletal	Arthrogryposis Cutaneous syndactyly Camptodactyly Radioulnar synostosis Osseous syndactyly Clinodactyly Hemangioma Lymphangioma Neurofibroma Enchondroma
III. Duplication	—	Whole limb Humerus Radius Ulna Digit	Mirror hand Polydactyly
IV. Overgrowth (gigantism)	—	Whole limb Partial limb Digit	Hemihypertrophy Macrodactyly
V. Undergrowth (hypoplasia)	—	Whole limb Whole hand Metacarpal Digit	Brachysyndactyly Brachydactyly
VI. Constriction band syndrome	Focal Amputation	—	Constriction band Acrosyndactyly Intrauterine amputation
VII. Generalized	—	—	Achondroplasia Marfan's syndrome

This table presents selected example diagnoses only, without subclassification. Some diagnoses can be conceivably placed in more than one category. For example, Swanson noted that brachysyndactyly (symbrachydactyly) could be placed in category I, II, or V.

hand are examples of category III congenital differences.

Category IV, "overgrowth," is subcategorized based on the anatomic area involved and includes hemihypertrophy and macrodactyly. Category V, "undergrowth," includes hypoplasia and brachydactyly. Category VI, "constriction band syndrome," consists of a wide array of clinical findings attributable to constricting amniotic rings, ranging from mild skin invaginations to complete amputations. Finally, category VII consists of "generalized skeletal abnormalities" and includes various forms of dwarfism and osteogenesis imperfecta, for example.

Modifications and Other Classification Systems

Since its inception, several modifications of the Swanson/IFSSH classification system have been proposed. One of the most significant suggested modifications is that of the Japanese Society for Surgery of the Hand (JSSH) and concerns cleft hand deformity, syndactyly, and polydactyly.[27,28] The JSSH modification highlights the limitations of the current Swanson/IFSSH classification and also demonstrates the difficulties encountered when attempting to alter it.

In typical cleft hand, in addition to suppression or absence of the central rays, central polydactyly and syndactyly are often present. Furthermore, clinical observation and recent embryologic studies support a common etiology for central polydactyly, syndactyly, and typical cleft hand.[27,28] Syndactyly and polydactyly are not grouped with typical cleft hand in the Swanson/ISSH classification, however. Cleft hand is classified under failure of formation (category I), syndactyly is categorized under failure of differentiation (category II), and central polydactyly falls under duplication (category III). This has led the JSSH to propose a new category that includes all these anomalies under the heading "abnormal induction of digital rays" (**Table 2**).[29] Although this makes sense from an embryologic standpoint, the new category separates radial and ulnar polydactyly from central polydactyly, resulting in the separation of morphologically similar congenital hand differences.

Another difficulty arose with the issue of symbrachydactyly and atypical cleft hand. Atypical cleft hand is now known to be a special instance of symbrachydactyly (oligodactylic symbrachydactyly). In the original Swanson/IFSSH classification, atypical cleft hand was classified under failure of formation in category I, whereas symbrachydactyly was categorized as undergrowth in category V. In most current modifications of the Swanson/IFSSH classification system, symbrachydactyly is brought up to category I and replaces or is placed beside the older term *atypical cleft hand*.[28,30] It is interesting to note that Swanson recognized that symbrachydactyly could be considered a failure of formation even though he placed it in the undergrowth category because of its primary morphologic presentation (hypoplasia).[23] This highlights the fact that the Swanson/IFSSH classification is truly morphologically and not etiologically based. In fact, as our understanding of embryology and teratology increases, it becomes more evident that a morphologically based classification system, although clinically useful, may not be embryologically correct.

Finally, a multitude of classification systems exist for grading specific congenital hand differences, such as those for thumb deficiency, radial longitudinal deficiency, and syndactyly.[31–33] These classification systems are often based on grade of severity or severity of expression and can be quite useful because of implications for prognosis and treatment. These classification systems are discussed elsewhere in this issue.

SUMMARY

The genetic and molecular bases for the embryologic development of the limb and for congenital hand differences are just beginning to be understood. Future investigations are likely to advance our understanding of the etiology of these problems and to influence the development of new modalities of intervention. The Swanson/IFSSH classification system is currently the basis for common discussion and study of congenital hand differences. Although this is quite difficult, future classification systems are likely to attempt

Table 2
Abbreviated Japanese Society for Surgery of the Hand modification

Main Category	Example
I. Failure of formation	Symbrachydactyly
II. Failure of differentiation	Radioulnar synostosis
III. Duplication	Radial polydactyly, ulnar polydactyly, mirror hand
IV. Abnormal induction of digital rays	Cutaneous syndactyly, osseous syndactyly, central polydactyly, typical cleft hand
V. Overgrowth	Macrodactyly
VI. Undergrowth	Brachydactyly, clinodactyly
VII. Constriction band syndrome	Constriction band
VIII. Generalized skeletal	Achondroplasia
IX. Others	—

to incorporate our rapidly increasing understanding of the genetic and molecular bases of these problems.

REFERENCES

1. Giele H, Giele C, Bower C, et al. The incidence and epidemiology of congenital upper limb anomalies: a total population study. J Hand Surg [Am] 2001; 26(4):628–34.
2. Bod M, Czeizel A, Lenz W. Incidence at birth of different types of limb reduction abnormalities in Hungary 1975–1977. Hum Genet 1983;65(1):27–33.
3. Kallen B, Rahmani TM, Winberg J. Infants with congenital limb reduction registered in the Swedish Register of Congenital Malformations. Teratology 1984;29(1):73–85.
4. Temtamy SA, McKusick VA. The genetics of hand malformations. Birth Defects Orig Artic Ser 1978; 14(3):i–xviii, 1–619.
5. Kozin S. Embryology. In: Green D, Hotchkiss R, Pederson W, et al, editors, Green's operative hand surgery, vol. 2. 5th edition. Philadelphia: Elsevier; 2005. p. 1375–9.
6. Daluiski A, Yi SE, Lyons KM. The molecular control of upper extremity development: implications for congenital hand anomalies. J Hand Surg [Am] 2001;26(1):8–22.
7. Netscher DT, Baumholtz MA. Treatment of congenital upper extremity problems. Plast Reconstr Surg 2007;119(5):101e–29e.
8. Mrazkova O. Ontogenesis of arterial trunks in the human fore-arm. Folia Morphol (Praha) 1973;21(2): 193–6.
9. Borud L, Upton J. Embryology of the upper limb. In: Hentz V, Mathes S, editors. Plastic surgery, vol. 8. Philadelphia: Saunders; 2006. p. 3–23.
10. Niswander L, Martin GR. Fgf-4 expression during gastrulation, myogenesis, limb and tooth development in the mouse. Development 1992;114(3):755–68.
11. Niswander L, Martin GR. FGF-4 and BMP-2 have opposite effects on limb growth. Nature 1993; 361(6407):68–71.
12. Niswander L, Tickle C, Vogel A, et al. FGF-4 replaces the apical ectodermal ridge and directs outgrowth and patterning of the limb. Cell 1993; 75(3):579–87.
13. Tickle C. Molecular basis of limb development. Biochem Soc Trans 1994;22(3):565–9.
14. Riddle RD, Tabin C. How limbs develop. Sci Am 1999;280(2):74–9.
15. Chiang C, Litingtung Y, Lee E, et al. Cyclopia and defective axial patterning in mice lacking Sonic hedgehog gene function. Nature 1996;383(6599): 407–13.
16. Laufer E, Nelson CE, Johnson RL, et al. Sonic hedgehog and Fgf-4 act through a signaling cascade and feedback loop to integrate growth and patterning of the developing limb bud. Cell 1994;79(6):993–1003.
17. Parr BA, McMahon AP. Dorsalizing signal Wnt-7a required for normal polarity of D-V and A-P axes of mouse limb. Nature 1995;374(6520):350–3.
18. Loomis CA, Kimmel RA, Tong CX, et al. Analysis of the genetic pathway leading to formation of ectopic apical ectodermal ridges in mouse Engrailed-1 mutant limbs. Development 1998; 125(6):1137–48.
19. Tickle C. Molecular basis of vertebrate limb patterning. Am J Med Genet 2002;112(3):250–5.
20. Muragaki Y, Mundlos S, Upton J, et al. Altered growth and branching patterns in synpolydactyly caused by mutations in HOXD13. Science 1996; 272(5261):548–51.
21. Mortlock DP, Innis JW. Mutation of HOXA13 in hand-foot-genital syndrome. Nat Genet 1997;15(2): 179–80.
22. Del Campo M, Jones MC, Veraksa AN, et al. Monodactylous limbs and abnormal genitalia are associated with hemizygosity for the human 2q31 region that includes the HOXD cluster. Am J Hum Genet 1999;65(1):104–10.
23. Swanson AB, Swanson GD, Tada K. A classification for congenital limb malformation. J Hand Surg [Am] 1983;8(5 Pt 2):693–702.
24. Swanson AB. A classification for congenital limb malformations. J Hand Surg [Am] 1976;1(1):8–22.
25. Kozin S. Congenital disorders: classification and diagnosis. In: Berger R, Weiss A-P, editors, Hand surgery, vol. 2. 1st edition. Philadelphia: Lippincott Williams & Wilkins; 2004. p. 1405–23.
26. Swanson AB. A classification for congenital malformations of the hand. NJ Bull Acad Med 1964;10: 166–9.
27. Ogino T. Teratogenic relationship between polydactyly, syndactyly and cleft hand. J Hand Surg [Br] 1990;15(2):201–9.
28. Miura T, Nakamura R, Horii E. The position of symbrachydactyly in the classification of congenital hand anomalies. J Hand Surg [Br] 1994;19(3): 350–4.
29. Congenital Hand Committee of the JSSH. Modified IFSSH classification. Journal of Japanese Society for Surgery of the Hand 2000;17:353–65.
30. Manske PR. Symbrachydactyly instead of atypical cleft hand. Plast Reconstr Surg 1993;91(1):196.
31. Lourie GM, Lins RE. Radial longitudinal deficiency. A review and update. Hand Clin 1998;14(1): 85–99.
32. Eaton CJ, Lister GD. Syndactyly. Hand Clin 1990; 6(4):555–75.
33. Manske PR, McCarroll HR Jr, James M. Type III-A hypoplastic thumb. J Hand Surg [Am] 1995; 20(2):246–53.

Congenital Failure of Formation of the Upper Limb

Paul R. Manske, MD[a],*, Charles A. Goldfarb, MD[b]

KEYWORDS

- Congenital anomalies • Failure of formation
- Radial longitudinal deficiency
- Central longitudinal deficiency
- Ulnar longitudinal deficiency

Congenital failure of formation abnormalities are manifested as longitudinal deformities of the hand and upper extremity and represent developmental abnormalities of the embryonic limb bud.[1] The development of the limb bud proceeds along three axes. The proximal-distal axis is controlled by the apical epidermal ridge (AER) and underlying mesoderm through fibroblast growth factor. The anterior-posterior axis (referred to as radial-ulnar by hand surgeons) is controlled by the zone of polarized activity (ZPA) on the posterior border of the limb bud through a morphogen, sonic hedgehog. The dorsal-ventral axis is controlled by Wnt-7a located in the dorsal ectoderm. The AER and ZPA are linked by diffusion through a feedback loop; genetic abnormalities or teratogenic insults to these zones are likely responsible for the longitudinal failures of formation; the specific abnormalities relate to the dosage and gestational time of the insult.

RADIAL LONGITUDINAL DEFICIENCY

Radial longitudinal deficiency (RLD) includes a spectrum of osseous, musculotendinous, and neurovascular deficiencies of the radial border of upper limb. Classification of these abnormalities are organized according to specific deficiencies of radius and thumb. Radius deficiencies are frequently associated with skeletal abnormalities of the spine, feet, and lower limb, as well as hematologic (Thrombocytopenia-Absent Radius

syndrome), cardiac (Holt Oram syndrome), renal, and gastrointestinal (tracheoesophageal fistula, imperforate anus) abnormalities. It is important that these other potential abnormalities are also be evaluated, either by the hand surgeon or other qualified pediatricians or surgeons, using chest radiographs, cardiac and renal ultrasound, spinal radiographs, and a hematologic work-up (complete blood cell count and peripheral blood smear) at the time of the initial encounter.[2]

Radius Deficiency

Formerly known as radial club hand because of the angled position of the hand at the distal forearm, the condition is now more acceptably referred to as radius deficiency. The abnormal features extend well beyond the radius abnormalities and may include general hypoplasia of the upper extremity, absence of active elbow flexion, shortening and bowing of the ulna, absence or hypoplasia of the scaphoid, and other radial-sided carpal bones. In the hand, the thumb is always affected, and the fingers frequently have limited motion and function proceeding radial to ulnar.[3] The musculotendinous structures on the radial aspect of the forearm may be absent or aberrant, the tendons often forming an unyielding fibrous tether at the wrist which, along with the skeletal deficiency, contributes to the angled position of the hand. The wrist is also flexed because of the over pull of the

a Department of Orthopaedic Surgery, Washington University School of Medicine, 660 South Euclid Avenue, Campus Box 8233, St. Louis, MO 63110, USA
b Department of Orthopaedic Surgery, Washington University School of Medicine at Barnes Jewish Hospital, 660 South Euclid Avenue, Campus Box 8233, St. Louis, MO 63110, USA
* Corresponding author.
E-mail address: manskep@wudosis.wustl.edu (P.R. Manske).

Hand Clin 25 (2009) 157–170
doi:10.1016/j.hcl.2008.10.005
0749-0712/08/$ – see front matter

extrinsic flexor muscles relative to the more hypoplastic extensor muscles.

Bayne and Klug[4] initially classified four types of radius deficiency (**Fig. 1**): type I, "short" distal radius; type II, hypoplastic radius "in miniature"; type III, absent distal radius; and type IV, complete absent radius. Types III and IV represent the most severe form of radius deficiency. James and colleagues[5] expanded the classification to include deficiencies of the radial carpal bones with a normal length distal radius as type 0, and isolated thumb abnormalities as type N. They also defined type I more specifically as a distal radius with more than 2 mm shortening with respect to the distal ulna.

Recently, Goldfarb and colleagues[6] proposed type V, proximal RLD, which includes manifestations in the proximal upper extremity and has the following characteristics: abnormal

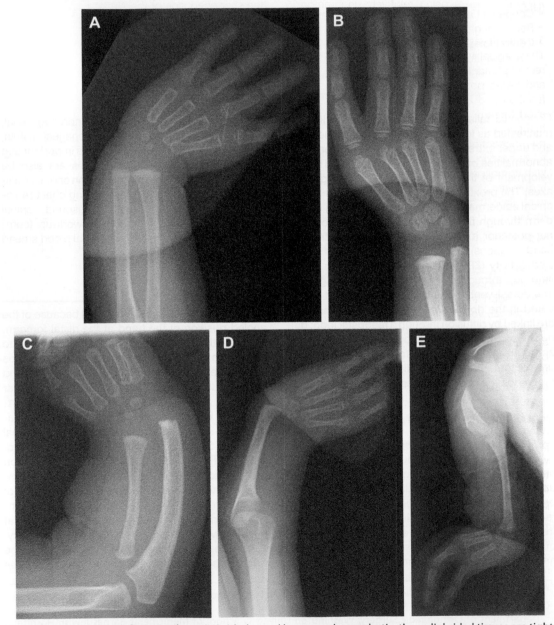

Fig. 1. (*A*) Type 0 radius deficiency. The radial-sided carpal bones are hyposplastic; the radial-sided tissues are tight; the thumb is absent. (*B*) Type I radius deficiency. The radius is more than 2 cm shorter than the ulna and the hand radially deviated. (*C*) Type II radius deficiency. The radius is hypoplastic ("radius in miniature"). (*D*) Type IV radius deficiency. The radius is completely absent. (*E*) Type V radius deficiency. Abnormal glenoid, absent proximal humerus, distal humerus articulates with ulna, radial-sided hand abnormalities.

glenoid, absent proximal humerus, distal humerus articulates with ulna, radial-sided hand abnormalities. This condition was formerly considered to be a form of phocomelia. However, the concept of an intercalary segmental defect is difficult to explain from a developmental biology perspective, and the concept of phocomelia has been challenged.[6,7] Instead, the several forms of phocomelia have been proposed to represent more severe forms of RLD and ulnar longitudinal deficiencies (ULD).[6]

Surgical treatment

The surgical treatment of radius deficiency is directed primarily to correcting the radial angulation and flexed position of the carpus to improve the function and appearance of the hand. While the short forearm also is a major limitation to normal function, perhaps more so than the angulated carpus, distraction lengthening of the ulna using an external fixator is an arduous procedure and fraught with complications.[8–10] Although increased length is obtained, the forearm does not equal that of the contralateral side and the decreased girth of the forearm due to undeveloped musculature remains.

Type 0 Not all type 0 hands require surgery; only those with notable angulation of more than 20° and lack of active extension to the neutral position. Mo and Manske[11] described soft tissue releases and tendon transfers to address this condition. The dorsal, volar, and radial wrist capsule are released, along with the tight insertions of the extensor carpi radialis longus and extensor carpi radialis brevis tendons (both may not always be present), to allow passive ulnar deviation of the wrist to the neutral position or beyond. The radial wrist extensors are then transferred to the distal stump of the extensor carpi ulnaris (ECU) tendon to enhance active ulnar deviation, and the detached proximal ECU tendon is transferred to the dorsal wrist capsule at the base of the third metacarpal to obtain wrist extension. This procedure averaged 46° improvement in ulnar deviation and 54° improvement in wrist extension.

Type I In addition to the short distal radius, the radial wrist extensors and capsular structures are also tight, as in type 0. Consequently, soft tissue release as described above is in order, along with the described tendon transfers. Additionally, in the authors' experience, the distal radius can be lengthened up to 20 mm by callotasis distraction using an external fixator to achieve an equal length of the distal radius and ulna.

Type II Little has been written about surgical correction of type II radius deficiency. The radius "in miniature" is often associated with marked bowing of the radius. Distraction lengthening of the ulna has been reported in two patients and we have lengthened the radius in a single stage on two occasions with improved results.[12]

Types III and IV Operative procedures have been performed most frequently to address the absence of the entire radius or the distal portion. There are two treatment concepts. The first is to release the tight radial soft structures and place the hand and carpus on the distal ulna; this is known as centralization. The other is to reconstruct an osseous support on the radial side of the wrist using microvascular tissue transfer of the metatarsal phalangeal joint from the foot.

The centralization procedure includes three components: precentralization soft tissue stretching; realignment and stabilization of the carpal bones on the distal ulna; and balancing the potentially deforming forces by tendon transfer and correction of the ulna bow.

Traditionally, the precentralization stretching of the soft tissues was accomplished by serial casting of the infant's wrist, correcting the ulnar angulation, and aligning the wrist with the distal end of the ulna. The serial casting was instituted shortly after birth and continued until the centralization procedure was performed. While the cast can correct the abnormal angulation, it does not effectively distract the tight radial soft tissues to allow placement of the carpus on the end of the distal ulna. Consequently, in recent years, distraction of the tight radial tissues has been accomplished more effectively using an external fixator for 6 to 8 weeks before performing the centralization procedure **(Fig. 2)**.[13,14] The precentralization soft tissue distraction not only improves the angulation of the deviated hand but also distracts the hand distally. In a recent series, the hand forearm angle was corrected 80°; the hand position was improved 29 mm ulnarward with respect to the ulna; and the volar subluxation of the carpus was corrected to the neutral position before the centralization procedure.[13] The improvement in position made the subsequent centralization technically easier to perform.

The second component of centralization by aligning the carpal bones on the distal end of the ulna was initially described in 1893 by Sayre[15] and numerous subsequent authors, using a variety of different surgical incisions.[16–26] The tight soft tissues on the radial side of the carpus are again released dorsally, volarly, and radially to allow transposition of the carpus onto the distal ulna. The distal ulna is frequently enlarged relative to the carpus, and the wrist and hand are unstable

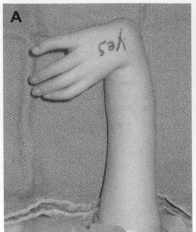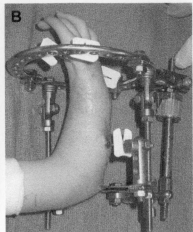

Fig. 2. (*A*) Type IV radius deficiency with severe radial deviation of the hand. (*B*) Precentralization soft tissue distraction with circular external fixator frame.

as they are perched on the distal ulna. It is important that the carpus is easily positioned on the distal ulna without soft tissue tension to prevent recurrence of the deformity. The precentralization soft tissue distraction has been most effective in addressing this issue. However, at times additional procedures must be performed to reduce the tension, particularly if preoperative soft tissue distraction has not been performed. These include: trimming the soft tissue and cartilage at the distal ulna, taking care not to injure the distal ulna physis; excision of the proximal carpal bones; and reduction osteotomy of the more proximal ulna diaphysis. The wrist and hand are stabilized on the ulna with a heavy K-wire for an extended period of time, up to 6 months.

The third component of centralization is to attempt to balance the deforming forces on the aligned hand and carpus. Buck-Gramcko[17] advocated "radialization;" that is, placement of the distal ulna to the radial side of the carpus to improve the mechanical stability of the hand on the distal end of the ulna; the long-term results of this procedure are not available. Additionally, various authors have recommended tendon transfers to the ulnar side of the hand and carpus to prevent recurrence of radial deviation. These include advancing the insertion of the ECU tendon to provide an ulnar and dorsal force to the wrist and hand.[4,23,24,27] Other suggested transfers to the base of the fifth metacarpal include: ring flexor digitorum superficialis and the common radial flexor and extensor muscles on the radial side of the wrist.[17,28] Our preferred transfer is the advancement of the ECU tendon. Additionally, at the time of centralization, we also redirect the radial vector of the extensor tendons (which pull from their origin on the lateral

epicondyle) to a longitudinal vector paralleling the course of the ulna using a soft tissue sling from a strip of the extensor reticulum at the time of the initial dissection. Finally, the abnormal radial vector of the extensor musculature is magnified by an ulnar bow when present. Corrective osteotomy of the ulnar bow is used whenever possible to reduce this radial directed vector.

Results

Centralization of the carpus on the ulna is an unstable construct. In the normal wrist, the carpus rests between two supporting proximal structures, the radius and ulna. In the postcentralized wrist, the single bony support for the carpus is highly unstable. Consequently, it is not surprising that after centralization, the hand does not always remain aligned at the end of the ulna. All reports indicate improvement following centralization, but not complete correction, of the radial deviation with continued loss of correction with time.[18–22,24] Additionally, the centralization procedure focuses on correcting the radial deviation; it does not effectively address wrist flexion. Consequently, wrist flexion frequently reoccurs, albeit not to the extent that it was pre-operatively.

Furthermore, there is evidence that centralization potentially impairs the growth of the distal ulna physis, particularly if the carpal bones need to be resected to get the hand and carpus at the end of the distal ulna.[29] This observation was made before the use of precentralization distraction, and the impact of this preliminary procedure on growth of the distal ulna physis is not known.

Perhaps the procedure that most affectively stabilizes the wrist and improves the aesthetic appearance of the forearm and hand is wrist arthrodesis, or epiphyseal arthrodesis in the case of skeletally immature patients.[30,31] Although many consider arthrodesis as a salvage procedure for failed centralization, the authors feel strongly it should be considered the definitive procedure for types III and IV radius deficient wrists in adolescence and adults. We advise parents that centralization should be viewed as the first stage of a potential two stage arthrodesis; we have performed epiphyseal arthrodesis in 11 patients with excellent success (unpublished data).

Historically, several attempts have been made to reconstruct radial support using a nonvascularized free fibular graft or the proximal part of the fibula.[32,33] However, these attempts failed because the grafted component did not grow. Vilkki[34] performed free vascularized tissue transfer of the second metatarsal phalangeal joint as an articulated radial support structure and reported excellent early results. However, in the ensuing 10 years, there have been no subsequent reports by Vilkki or other authors. Despite its conceptual appeal, free vascularized transfer of a radial sided support has not been popularly adopted.

Hypoplastic Thumb

The hypoplastic thumb can occur as an isolated entity or in conjunction with any of the radius deficiencies noted above. The classification includes five categories that reflect the progressive stages of arrested development.[35] The features of each category are well defined, particularly types II, IV, and V. The more subtle manifestations of types I and II hypoplastic thumb may go unrecognized by parents and referring pediatricians, especially in the presence of more obvious manifestations of radial longitudinal deficiency in the opposite extremity. It is incumbent on the hand surgeon to carefully examine both hands of any child presenting with RLD.

Classification

Type I The thumb may be decreased in size. The intrinsic abductor pollicis brevis (ABP) and opponents pollicis (OP) musculature is hypoplastic or absent.[36]

Type II There are three specific features: narrowing of the thumb-index web space; aplasia or hypoplasia of the APB and OP intrinsic muscles sparing the flexor pollicis brevis (FPB) and adductor pollicis (AddP) muscles; and instability of the ulnar collateral ligament at the metacarpophalangeal (MP) joint. The narrowed thumb web space and unstable ulnar collateral ligament interfere with the child's ability to pinch or grasp objects. The deficiency of the intrinsic muscles of opposition interferes with the child's ability to rotate the thumb in front of the fingers and thereby contributes to ineffective pinch.

Type III The three manifestations of type II thumb hypoplasia are also present in type III, often in more severe form. The narrowed thumb-index web space may present as a more distal take-off of the thumb from the hand; the MP instability may be more global, also involving the radial collateral ligament. Additionally, there are two other potential deficiencies: abnormalities of the extrinsic muscles or tendons and osseous deficiencies of the thumb metacarpal base.[37] The most frequently observed extrinsic musculotendinous abnormalities include: absent extensor pollicis longus (EPL), absent or aberrant flexor pollicis longus (FPL), and tendon interconnections between the flexor and extensor tendons—either in the digit itself or more proximally in the thenar area or distal forearm.[37,38] The so called pollex abductus thumb, described by Tupper[39] is a form of type III thumb hypoplasia.

In type III-A hypoplasia, the carpal metacarpal joint is present and stable, although the thumb metacarpal base may be hypoplastic. In type III-B hypoplasia, the thumb metacarpal base is absent and the carpal metacarpal joint is unstable.[37]

Type IV Type IV hypoplasia is the classic pouce flottant: the thumb is attached to the hand only by a narrow soft tissue skin bridge containing neurovascular elements. There are no musculotendinous structures or osseous elements joining the thumb to the hand.

Type V Type V hypoplasia represents complete absence of the thumb. However, there may be rudimentary thenar muscles, tendons, or neurovascular structures along the radial border of the index metacarpal.

Surgical treatment

Reconstruction of the hypoplastic thumb Reconstruction of the hypoplastic thumb is indicated for types I, II, and III-A. The narrow thumb-index web space can be widened by standard 3-, 4- or 5-flap Z-plasties. The procedure should also include release of the fascia investing the AddP and first dorsal interosseous muscles. On infrequent occasion, the origin of these muscles must be released from the bone and advanced to facilitate widening of the thumb-index space.

Stabilization of the MP joint is essential to enhance the function of the hypoplastic thumb. In children, this can usually be accomplished by imbricating the ulnar capsule at the MP joint and reinforcing it with distal end of the tendon used for the opposition transfer. When the radial collateral ligament of the thumb is also deficient (as seen in the more severe type III-A hypoplasia), stabilization of both the radial capsule and ulnar capsule by imbrication may be attempted. However, this may not result in adequate stabilization and metacarpophalangeal epiphyseal arthrodesis of the MP joint, which preserves the growth plate, may be necessary.[40]

An opposition transfer using either the abductor digiti minimi or the flexor digitorum superficialis of the ring finger is necessary to restore opposition function.[41,42] We prefer the abductor digiti minimi transfer described originally by Huber[43] and by Nicholaysen[44] (**Fig. 3**). This is a muscle transfer, rather than a tendon transfer; consequently, an adequate subcutaneous tunnel needs to be developed across the palm to accommodate the transposed muscle. We prefer to leave the muscle origin attached to the pisiform as originally described by Huber and Nicholaysen, because this osseous origin is thought to be a source of vascularization for the muscle.[45] We prefer this over detaching the muscle origin as described by Littler and Cooley.[46]

Extrinsic tendon deficiencies must be considered in the surgical reconstruction of type III-A hypoplastic thumbs.[37] Not all extrinsic tendon abnormalities require surgical treatment; only those that limit function or result in aesthetically displeasing deformities. The most straightforward procedure is the release of tendon and muscle interconnections that cause deformities or limit motion. We prefer to limit releases to the thumb itself (eg, interconnections between the extensor aponeurosis and the FPL, release of the aberrant FPL tendon insertion that radially deviates the thumb), but others advocate exploration of the thenar area and distal forearm to release deforming musculotendinous interconnections.[38]

An absent EPL tendon limits thumb extension and is a substantial limitation to function. It can be treated with extensor indicis proprius transfer. An absent FPL limits IP flexion; it can be addressed by one of several methods: rerouting the aberrant FPL tendon to a more volar position on the thumb, transferring the ring finger superficialis tendon to the distal phalanx, or accepting the slight functional limitation of absent IP joint flexion and relying on the intrinsic FPB musculature to flex the MP joint.

Shibata and colleagues[47] described converting type III-B thumbs to III-A thumbs by transferring a vascularized metatarsal phalangeal joint to the base of the thumb in four patients. This procedure allows preservation of thumbs when cultural aesthetics encourage a five digit hand.

Index finger pollicization Absent or nonfunctioning type III-B, IV or V thumbs are treated by excision and pollicization of the index finger, rotating the index ray on its neurovascular pedicle to the position of the thumb.[48–51] The procedure has three primary objectives: improve the ability to grasp large objects; improve the appearance (ie, a hand with a thumb and three fingers is a less noticeably abnormality than a four-fingered hand without a thumb); and facilitating hand shakes when the right hand is involved. Pollicization is preferable to free vascularized tissue transfer of a toe to the hand because the proximal osseous, musculocutaneous, and neurovascular structures necessary

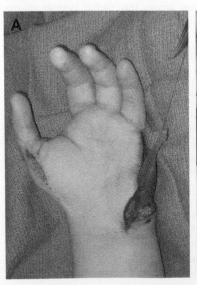 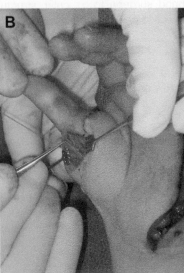

Fig. 3. (*A*) Abductor digiti minimi opposition transfer. (*B*) Abductor digiti minimi muscle transposed subcutaneously across the palm to the thumb.

for such transfer are not present in patients who have congenital aplasia of the thumb. The function of the pollicized digit is related to the pre-operative condition of the index finger, which has varying degrees of joint motion and tendon excursion. An index finger with severe limitations should not be pollicized.

The timing of the operation is controversial. While it has been recommended that pollicization be performed before 12 months (when cortical representation and awareness of the thumb develop in a normal child), we feel that the index finger is cortically represented as the radial post in a child with an absent or nonfunctioning thumb.[48] Therefore, results of the operative repositioning of the index ray should not be related to age. A long-term study of pollicizations performed between the ages of 9 months and 16 years showed no differences in function related to age at operation.[52] Early operative intervention may be encouraged for social reasons related to restoration of the normal appearance of the hand as early as possible, rather than for enhancing the cortical representation of the pollicized digit as a thumb or for maximizing function.

The technical aspects of pollicization have been well described following the principles well outlined by Buck-Gramcko.[48] These include: skin incision, skeletal shortening by removing the index metacarpal shaft, digital rotation, and transfer of the first dorsal and volar intrinsic muscles to provide abductor and adductor function.[48–51] Skin closure to give the pollicized digit the appearance of a thumb, rather than a finger in the position of the thumb, is an important technical consideration (**Fig. 4**). This can be accomplished by attaching the skin web from the adjacent long finger at the level of the proximal interphalangeal (PIP) joint of the pollicized digit (ie, "MP joint" of the "new thumb"), rather than at the MP joint of the pollicized digit (ie, "carpometacarpal joint" of the "new thumb").

In general, the results of pollicization have been good as reported by several authors.[42,48,50,52,53] In our experience, there has been no evidence of altered sensibility of the pollicized digit, and all patients used the pollicized digit for activities. All patients used the pollicized digit for grasping large objects. However, patients who used the long-ring or ring-small interspace to grasp and manipulate small objects preoperatively, continued to do so postoperatively.

In a more detailed study the pollicized digit had approximately 50% the range of motion of a normal thumb.[52] It was used for 85% of activities, particularly for grasping large objects.

Performance of activities as measured by the Jebsen-Taylor Hand Function Test took 22% longer to perform than did activities performed with a normal hand.[54] Function was near normal when the pollicized index finger had minimum deficiency; more deficient index fingers, such as those seen in conjunction with more severe proximal manifestations or RLD, had reduced function. Clark and colleagues[53] reported similar generally good results, particularly in patients with preoperative isolated thumb aplasia.

Reduced strength is the most noticeable functional deficiency of the pollicized digit. Clark and

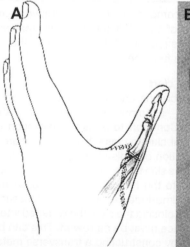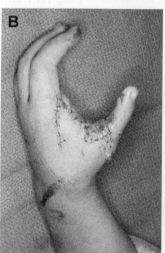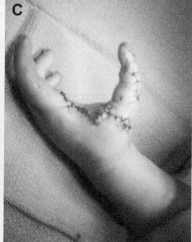

Fig. 4. (*A*) Drawing of attachment of skin web from the adjacent long finger to the pollicized digit at the level of the PIP joint to give appearance of a thumb. (*B*) Pollicized digit with appearance of a thumb. (*C*) Pollicized digit with appearance of a finger in the position of the thumb.

colleagues[53] noted strength was greater than 50% of the opposite thumb in isolated thumb aplasia, whereas the strength of pollicized digits associated with radius deficiency was less than 50% of the opposite thumb. Manske and colleagues[52] noted even greater reduction in grip and pinch strength, reporting 33% of normal thumb values in patients with minimal index finger deficiencies and 15% of normal thumb values in patients with more severe manifestations of RLD. The authors attribute the weakness of the pollicized digit primarily to a weak intrinsic adductor function. In the normal hand, the AddP is a substantial muscle with a large force vector pulling the thumb toward the palm. In contrast, the adductor function of the pollicized digit is accomplished by the transferred first volar interosseous muscle, a relatively weak muscle with a vector of pull in the pollicized digit, which is not directed into the palm.

CENTRAL LONGITUDINAL DEFICIENCY

Central longitudinal deficiency (CLD) is also known descriptively as cleft hand. The deficiency is characterized by varying degrees of suppression of the bones and associated soft tissue structures of the central hand. Although a soft tissue cleft alone can occur, the defect usually includes varying degrees of suppression of the central rays.[55,56] In its most severe form, the thumb is also suppressed. The defect does not extend proximal to the wrist, although carpal coalition and radial ulnar synostosis are sometimes associated with central deficiency.[55] Central deficiency occurs in association with central polydactyly and osseous syndactyly.[57–59] There is little functional deficit related to the cleft itself.[60] The primary functional limitation is related to the thumb-index web space, which is narrowed to varying degrees.[61] Of interest, this progressive narrowing of the thumb web space parallels the progressive deficiencies of the central cleft.

Classification

Several classification systems have been proposed based on the characteristics of the central cleft. Barsky[62] initially distinguished between the typical cleft hand (deficiencies of the central rays with preservation of the marginal digits) and the atypical cleft hand (central rays of progressively reduced in size with shortened marginal digits). The current prevailing opinion is that the atypical cleft hand represents symbrachydactyly, a form of transverse deficiency, and, therefore, is not a component of CLDs.[57,63] Other authors have classified the cleft according to whether central polydactyly and osseous syndactyly is present;

the associated central polydactyly and osseous syndactyly was also confusingly referred to as atypical cleft hands.[58,64] Finally, several authors classified hands according to the number of central osseous elements that are absent.[55,56,59,65]

As noted, the narrowed thumb web space represents a notable functional deficiency. Consequently, Manske and Halikis[61] proposed this classification of the central deficient hand based on the progressive narrowing of the thumb web space:

Type I. Normal web. There is no narrowing of the thumb web space.

Type II. Narrowed web. The thumb-index web space is narrowed, either mildly (type II-A) or severely (type II-B).

Type III. Syndactylized web. The thumb and index rays are syndactylized with complete obliteration of the web space. The index ray may be short with suppressed development of the middle phalanx.

Type IV. Merged web. The index ray is completely suppressed and the web space has merged with the cleft. Since the thumb functions effectively with the ulnar digits, this pattern is not functionally limiting. The ulnar collateral ligament at the MP joint may be deficient resulting in instability of the thumb.

Type V. Absent web. The thumb is no longer present; only the ulnar rays remain.

The value of this classification is that it can be used to guide operative treatment.

Surgical Treatment

There are two components to the operative treatment, closure of the cleft for aesthetic reasons and the reconstruction of the narrowed thumb web to improve function.

Closure of the cleft

Various skin incisions and local flaps have been proposed to accomplish closure of the cleft.[60,62,66,67] Common to all is the elevation of dorsal or palmar skin to close the intermetacarpal cleft and formation of a distal commissure. There is usually excess skin that should either be excised or transposed to the thumb web to increase the width of the thumb-index space when necessary.

In addition to closing the skin, the widened intermetacarpal space must be narrowed. This can be accomplished by constructing a transverse metacarpal ligament using local tissue flaps, such as the flexor tendon sheath from adjacent metacarpals, or placement of a circumferential tendon graft around the distal metacarpal necks. Alternatively, the intermetacarpal space may be narrowed by transposing the index ray ulnarward. As a general rule, reconstruction of the transverse metacarpal ligament is used for the less severe types I and II-A deficiencies; whereas transposition of the index metacarpal is used for the more severely narrowed types II-B and III deficiencies.

Thumb web space reconstruction

The techniques for reconstructing the thumb web space vary according to the type of central deficiency. In the mild type II-A deficiencies, local 3-, 4- or 5-flap Z-plasties are usually effective.[68,69]

However, the available local skin is usually insufficient to adequately widen the severely narrowed web space seen in type II-B deficiencies. Therefore, a dorsal or palmar pedicle flap is transposed from the cleft into the web space.[70,71] Split thickness skin grafts may also be needed to cover open areas. We prefer to transpose dorsal flaps, because it is more important for adequate thumb function to have sufficient pliable skin on the dorsal aspect of web space than on the palmar side (**Fig. 5**). At times, both dorsal and volar flaps must be used. Ulnar transposition of the index ray is also frequently performed to facilitate widening of the web space.

Type III thumb-index syndactyly deficiencies are technically challenging and the most difficult web spaces to reconstruct. The primary objective is to reconstruct the thumb web space. However, if the index ray is too short, it should be excised, thus forming a merged space (ie, type IV).

Reconstruction involves separation of the syndactyly, in addition to formation of the web space. While staging the operation has been proposed, initially releasing the syndactyly digit and reconstructing the web later, most surgeons prefer to accomplish both procedures in a single operation.[72] The syndactyly digits are released in standard fashion using skin grafts as necessary to fill the covered areas. Both palmar and dorsal base flaps are frequently needed to reconstruct the web space along with ulnar transposition of the index ray. Of note, the thumb and index extensor and flexor tendons may be commonly joined and must be separated longitudinally. Unfortunately, they frequently have a common muscle, and independent function of the thumb and index finger will be limited. The middle phalanx of the index finger is often short and delta-shaped, thus creating a radial digit deviated toward the thumb following syndactyly separation.

Severe type II-B and III cleft deformities often include an infrequently reported flexion contracture of the ring finger PIP joint or the digit is rotated in supination. The deformity is likely due to the congenitally deficient radial sided intrinsic muscles (ie, the third lumbrical and second volar interosseous) of the ring finger. Because of the intrinsic muscle deficiencies, the PIP joint has no active extension in utero, which results in a flexion contracture; the unopposed ulnar intrinsic muscles rotate the digit. We have not attempted to obtain PIP joint extension using tendon transfers, but have treated the rotational deformity by corrective osteotomy of the proximal phalanx.

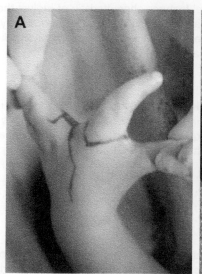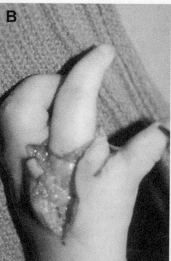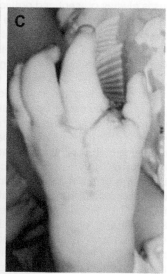

Fig. 5. (*A*) Type II-B central deficiency hand with severe narrowing of thumb-index web space. (*B*) Type II-B central deficiency hand with severe narrowing of thumb-index web space which is widened by transposition of dorsal flap from the cleft. (*C*) Postoperative transposition of dorsal flap from cleft to widen thumb-index web space.

Operative procedures for the type IV merged thumb web and cleft are frequently not necessary; the increased distance between the thumb and ulnar digits is usually not a functional problem. Excess skin in the web space can be excised as necessary. Instability of the MP joint ulnar collateral ligament may require capsular imbrication in young children or epiphyseal arthrodesis to stabilize the thumbs of older children.[40]

Type V deficiencies are infrequently seen. Kay and Wiberg[73] have performed toe to hand free tissue transfer to provide an oppositional post for the monodactylous small finger. However, this procedure must be performed with caution because the proximal anatomic structures may not be present in central deficiency, and patients may have central foot deficiencies that preclude transposition of the toes.

ULNAR LONGITUDINAL DEFICIENCY

ULD represents a spectrum of abnormalities along the ulnar border of the limb. The incidence is less than for RLD or CLD. Although the deficiencies follow the ulnar longitudinal axis in the forearm and upper arm, both the ulnar and radial sides of the hand are affected. This discrepancy is likely explained by the location of the ZPA on the postaxial (ulnar) border of the limb bud. The ZPA produces the morphogen (sonic hedgehog) which, through concentration gradients, influences the development of the radial and ulnar aspects of the distal limb bud.[74–76]

The extremity is short and there is frequently limited elbow motion, due either to dislocation of the radial head or radial humeral synostosis. The radius is always present and provides a stable articulation for the carpal bones. The ulna is frequently absent or hypoplastic. The most notable ulna deformity is marked pronation or anterior bowing of the ulna that orients the hand in an internally rotated or posterior direction. A fibrocartilaginous anlage connecting the undeveloped ulna to the distal radius and carpal bones has been implicated in causing deformities of the forearm and wrist.[60,77–80] It may act as a tether resulting in decreased growth of the distal radial physis, ulnar deviation of the wrist, bowing of the radius, and dislocation of the radial head. Investigators have noted these deformities are relatively static when present.[81–84] Hand abnormalities are present in 68% to 100% of ULD extremities.[77,81,84–86] The deformities are varied and affect both the ulnar and radial sides of the hand. The deformities include absent digits, syndactylized digits, malrotated rays, hypoplastic tendons and muscles.

ULDs are classified according to both forearm-elbow deformities and hand deformities.

Classification

Forearm-elbow

Six similar classifications based on forearm-elbow deformities have been presented.[78,79,84,87–89] The four category classification of Bayne,[87] which parallels the classification of radius deficiencies, is generally preferred. Interestingly, none of the six forearm-elbow classifications includes hand abnormalities. Consequently, Bayne's ULD classification has recently been modified to include type 0, which recognizes the presence of hand abnormalities in the presence of a normal elbow and forearm.[90] Additionally, similar to the inclusion of phocomelia-type limbs as RLDs, proximal manifestations of ULD have been added to the classification as type V.[6] The classifications are:

Type 0. The ulna is of normal length with respect to the distal radius. The deficiencies are limited to the hand.

Type I. The ulna is hypoplastic and shortened but the distal and proximal epiphyses are present.

Type II. The distal portion of the ulna is aplastic.

Type III. The ulna is completely aplastic with the radius as the only forearm bone.

Type IV. The ulna is completely aplastic with there is synostosis of the radius and humerus (no elbow joint).

Type V. There are proximal manifestations of ULD, in addition to the distal deficiencies. The abnormalities include: hypoplastic glenoid, single arm or forearm bone with proximal features resembling a humerus and distal features characteristic of radius; the forearm bone is usually bifurcated distally; the elbow joint is absent; hand abnormalities are present typical of ULD.

Hand

Ogino and Kato[86] classified the hand abnormalities according the number of missing rays, proceeding sequentially from the ulnar to the radial side of the hand. The classification includes:

Type A. Absent small finger
Type B. Absent fifth ray
Type C. Absent fourth and fifth rays
Type D. Absent third, fourth and fifth rays
Type E. Absent second and fifth rays.

The classification does not include absence or abnormalities of the thumb. In the authors' experience the hand abnormalities do not follow an organized ulnar-radial sequential ectrodactyly pattern, but are more complex.

In view of the high incidence of thumb abnormalities and the importance of the thumb to the function of the hand, Cole and Manske[85] presented a classification scheme based on features of the thumb, suggesting the alphabetic letters be added to the roman numerals of the forearm-elbow classification views used by Bayne and others:

Type A. Normal first web and thumb
Type B. Mild first web and thumb deficiency
Type C. Moderate to severe first web deficiencies. These deficiencies include severe thumb or first web narrowing, thumb-index syndactyly, malrotation of the thumb in the plane of the other digits, hypoplasia of the thenar muscles, and absent extrinsic tendon function.
Type D. Absent thumb

Surgical Treatment

The above classification provides surgical guidance as to the relative incidence of operative procedures.[85] The number of operative procedures performed on both the forearm and the hands is greater in type C and D hands compared with type A and B hands. Grouping the procedures according to the forearm, thumb, first web, and other hand procedures, the number of surgical procedures for the thumb and first web exceeds the number of procedures for the forearm and the rest of the hand.

Forearm

Despite the obvious forearm deformities, patients with ulnar deficiency usually have few functional limitations and operative procedures are infrequently indicated. Although resection of the cartilaginous anlage has been advocated, it should not be resected unless it can be demonstrated that there is progressive ulnar deviation at the wrist, bowing of the radius, or dislocation of the radial head.

The most frequent forearm procedure is corrective osteotomy of the radius to address either the severe anterior bowing or the severe pronation deformity. The osteotomy places the forearm into a more neutral position so that the hand can be used in conjunction with the opposite uninvolved extremity.

Resection of a dislocated radial head can be performed for pain or an unsightly prominence.[91,92] However, resection is not frequently performed because the elbow is usually stable and functions well despite the dislocation.

Construction of a one bone forearm and fusion of the proximal radius and ulna has been proposed to treat forearm instability.[77,79,80,87,93] However, we have not encountered an unstable forearm in any ULD patient and therefore have not performed either of these procedures for this condition. We feel the soft tissues stabilize the deficient osseous structures in most cases.

Thumb or first web

Operative procedures for ULD extremities most frequently involve the thumb and thumb webspace.[85] The procedures include deepening of the thumb-index web space, release of the thumb-index syndactyly, rotational and abduction osteotomy of the thumb ray in the plane of the other digits, and reconstruction of a thumb-index web space using pedicle flaps. Other operative procedures include pollicization for an absent thumb, opposition transfer for thenar muscle hypoplasia, and epiphyseal arthrodesis for unstable MP or IP joints.

Other hand procedures

Hand procedures not involving the thumb include soft tissue syndactyly release, flexion contracture release, and rotational osteotomy of malformed digits.

While the above operative procedures have been considered beneficial to improving the function and aesthetics of patients with longitudinal deficiency, the number of reported cases is small and quantitative evaluation of the results have not been reported.

SUMMARY

In conclusion, longitudinal failure of formation deformities comprises a substantial portion of the anomalies of the upper limb. Although much of the past and current congenital hand literature has been devoted to these conditions, they continue to be a reconstructive challenge to hand surgeons involved in their care.

REFERENCES

1. Daluiski A, Yi SE, Lyons KM. The molecular control of upper extremity development: implications for congenital hand anomalies. J Hand Surg [Am] 2001; 26(1):8–22.
2. Goldfarb CA, Wall L, Manske PR. Radial longitudinal deficiency: the incidence of associated medical and musculoskeletal conditions. J Hand Surg [Am] 2006; 31(7):1176–82.
3. James MA, Green HD, McCarroll HR Jr, et al. The association of radial deficiency with thumb hypoplasia. J Bone Joint Surg Am 2004;86-A(10):2196–205.
4. Bayne LG, Klug MS. Long-term review of the surgical treatment of radial deficiencies. J Hand Surg [Am] 1987;12:169–79.

5. James MA, McCarroll HR Jr, Manske PR. The spectrum of radial longitudinal deficiency: a modified classification. J Hand Surg [Am] 1999;24(6): 1145–55.

6. Goldfarb CA, Manske PR, Busa R, et al. Upper-extremity phocomelia reexamined: a longitudinal dysplasia. J Bone Joint Surg Am 2005;87(12): 2639–48.

7. Tytherleigh-Strong G, Hooper G. The classification of phocomelia. J Hand Surg [Br] 2003;28:215–7.

8. Horii E, Nakamura R, Nakao E, et al. Distraction lengthening of the forearm for congenital and developmental problems. J Hand Surg [Br] 2000;25(1): 15–21.

9. Peterson BM, McCarroll HR Jr, James MA. Distraction lengthening of the ulna in children with radial longitudinal deficiency. J Hand Surg [Am] 2007; 32(9):1402–7.

10. Pickford MA, Scheker LR. Distraction lengthening of the ulna in radial club hand using the Ilizarov technique. J Hand Surg [Br] 1998;23(2):186–91.

11. Mo JH, Manske PR. Surgical treatment of type 0 radial longitudinal deficiency. J Hand Surg [Am] 2004;29(6):1002–9.

12. Matsuno T, Ishida O, Sunagawa T, et al. Radius lengthening for the treatment of Bayne and Klug type II and type III radial longitudinal deficiency. J Hand Surg [Am] 2006;31(5):822–9.

13. Goldfarb CA, Murtha YM, Gordon JE, et al. Soft-tissue distraction with a ring external fixator before centralization for radial longitudinal deficiency. J Hand Surg [Am] 2006;31(6):952–9.

14. Sabharwal S, Finuoli AL, Ghobadi F. Pre-centralization soft tissue distraction for Bayne type IV congenital radial deficiency in children. J Pediatr Orthop 2005;25(3):377–81.

15. Sayre RH. A contribution to the study of club-hand. Trans. Am Orthop Assn 1893;6:208–16.

16. Bora FW Jr, Nicholson JT, Cheema HM. Radial meromelia. The deformity and its treatment. J Bone Joint Surg Am 1970;52(5):966–79.

17. Buck-Gramcko D. Radialization as a new treatment for radial club hand. J Hand Surg [Am] 1985;10 (6 Pt 2):964–8.

18. Damore E, Kozin SH, Thoder JJ, et al. The recurrence of deformity after surgical centralization for radial clubhand. J Hand Surg [Am] 2000;25(4): 745–51.

19. Geck MJ, Dorey F, Lawrence JF, et al. Congenital radius deficiency: radiographic outcome and survivorship analysis. J Hand Surg [Am] 1999;24(6):1132–44.

20. Goldfarb CA, Klepps SJ, Dailey LA, et al. Functional outcome after centralization for radius dysplasia. J Hand Surg [Am] 2002;27(1):118–24.

21. Lamb DW. Radial club hand. A continuing study of sixty-eight patients with one hundred and seventeen club hands. J Bone Joint Surg Am 1977;59(1):1–13.

22. Lamb DW, Scott H, Lam WL, et al. Operative correction of radial club hand: a long-term follow-up of centralization of the hand on the ulna. J Hand Surg [Br] 1997;22:533–6.

23. Lidge RT. Congenital radial deficient club hand In Proceedings of the American Academy of Orthopaedic Surgeons. J Bone Joint Surg [Am] 1969;51:1041–2.

24. Manske PR, McCarroll HR Jr, Swanson K. Centralization of the radial club hand: an ulnar surgical approach. J Hand Surg [Am] 1981;6(5):423–33.

25. Skerick S, Flatt AE. The anatomy of congenital radial dysplasia. Its surgical and functional implications. Clin Orthop Relat Res 1969;66:125–43.

26. Watson HK, Beebe RD, Cruz NI. A centralization procedure for radial clubhand. J Hand Surg [Am] 1984;9(4):541–7.

27. Goldberg MJ, Meyn M. The radial clubhand. Orthop Clin North Am 1976;7(2):341–59.

28. Yamauchi Y. Vascularized epiphyseal transfers—animal experiments and some clinical experiences. Orthop Trans 1985;9:409.

29. Sestero AM, Van Heest A, Agel J. Ulnar growth patterns in radial longitudinal deficiency. J Hand Surg [Am] 2006;31(6):960–7.

30. Rayan GM. Ulnocarpal arthrodesis for recurrent radial clubhand deformity in adolescents. J Hand Surg [Am] 1992;17(1):24–7.

31. Cole RJ, Manske PR. Epiphyseal arthrodesis of the digital and wrist joints in children. Atlas of Hand Clinics 1998;3:161–78.

32. Albee FH. Formation of radius congenitally absent. Condition seven years after implantation of bone graft. Ann Surg 1928;87:105–10.

33. Starr DE. Congenital absence of the radius. A method of surgical correction. J Bone Joint Surg Am 1945;27:572–7.

34. Vilkki SK. Distraction and microvascular epiphysis transfer for radial club hand. J Hand Surg [Br] 1998;23(4):445–52.

35. Blauth W, Schneider-Sickert F. Numerical variations. In: Blauth W, Schneider-Sickert F, editors. Congenital deformities of the hand. An atlas on their surgical treatment. New York: Springer; 1981.

36. James MA, McCarroll HR Jr, Manske PR. Characteristics of patients with hypoplastic thumbs. J Hand Surg [Am] 1996;21(1):104–13.

37. Manske PR, McCarroll HR Jr, James M. Type III-A hypoplastic thumb. J Hand Surg [Am] 1995;20(2): 246–53.

38. Graham TJ, Louis DS. A comprehensive approach to surgical management of the type IIIA hypoplastic thumb. J Hand Surg [Am] 1998;23(1):3–13.

39. Tupper JW. Pollex abductus due to congenital malposition of the flexor pollicis longus. J Bone Joint Surg Am 1969;51:1285–90.

40. Kowalski MF, Manske PR. Arthrodesis of digital joints in children. J Hand Surg [Am] 1988;13(6):874–9.

41. Manske PR, McCarroll HR Jr. Abductor digiti minimi opponensplasty in congenital radial dysplasia. J Hand Surg [Am] 1978;3(6):552–9.

42. Lister G. Reconstruction of the hypoplastic thumb. Clin Orthop Relat Res 1985;(195):52–65.

43. Huber E. Hilfsoperation bei Medianuslahmung. Deutsche Zeitschr Chir 1921;162:271–5.

44. Nicholaysen J. Transplantation du muscle abducteur du petit doigt, dans un cas d'incapacite de mouvement d'opposition du ponce. Acta Chir Scand 1923;55:183–4.

45. Dunlap J, Manske PR, McCarthy JA. Perfusion of the abductor digiti quinti after transfer on a neurovascular pedicle. J Hand Surg [Am] 1989;14(6):992–5.

46. Littler JW, Cooley SGE. Opposition of the thumb and its restoration by abductor digiti quinti transfer. J Bone Joint Surg Am 1963;45:1389–96.

47. Shibata M, Yoshizu T, Seki T, et al. Reconstruction of a congenital hypoplastic thumb with use of a free vascularized metatarsophalangeal joint. J Bone Joint Surg Am 1998;80(10):1469–76.

48. Buck-Gramcko D. Pollicization of the index finger. Method and results in aplasia and hypoplasia of the thumb. J Bone Joint Surg Am 1971;53(8):1605–17.

49. Littler JW. The neurovascular pedicle method of digital transposition for reconstruction of the thumb. Plast Reconstr Surg 1953;12:303–19.

50. Manske PR, McCaroll HR Jr. Index finger pollicization for a congenitally absent or nonfunctioning thumb. J Hand Surg [Am] 1985;10(5):606–13.

51. Manske PR, McCarroll HR Jr. Reconstruction of the congenitally deficient thumb. Hand Clin 1992;8(1):177–96.

52. Manske PR, Rotman MB, Dailey LA. Long-term functional results after pollicization for the congenitally deficient thumb. J Hand Surg [Am] 1992;17(6):1064–72.

53. Clark DI, Chell J, Davis TR. Pollicisation of the index finger. A 27-year follow-up study. J Bone Joint Surg Br 1998;80(4):631–5.

54. Jebsen RH, Taylor N, Trieschmann RB, et al. An objective and standardised test of hand function. Arch Phys Med Rehabil 1969;50(6):311–9.

55. Nutt JN 3rd, Flatt AE. Congenital central hand deficit. J Hand Surg [Am] 1981;6(1):48–60.

56. Ogino T. Cleft hand. Hand Clin 1990;6(4):661–71.

57. Buck-Gramcko D. Cleft hands: classification and treatment. Hand Clin 1985;1(3):467–73.

58. Tada K, Yonenobu K, Swanson AB. Congenital central ray deficiency in the hand—a survey of 59 cases and subclassification. J Hand Surg [Am] 1981;6(5):434–41.

59. Watari S, Tsuge K. A classification of cleft hands, based on clinical findings: theory of development mechanism. Plast Reconstr Surg 1979;64:381–9.

60. Flatt AE. The care of congenital hand anomalies. St. Louis: C.V. Mosby; 1977.

61. Manske PR, Halikis MN. Surgical classification of central deficiency according to the thumb web. J Hand Surg [Am] 1995;20(4):687–97.

62. Barsky AJ. Cleft hand: classification, incidence, and treatment. review of the literature and report of nineteen cases. J Bone Joint Surg Am Dec 1964;46:1707–20.

63. Ogino T, Minami A, Kato H. Clinical features and roentgenograms of symbrachydactyly. J Hand Surg [Br] 1989;14:303–6.

64. Sandzen SC Jr. Classification and functional management of congenital central defect of the hand. Hand Clin 1985;1(3):483–98.

65. Saito H, Seki T, Suzuki Y, et al. Operative treatments for various types of the cleft hand. Seikei Geka 1978;29:1551–3.

66. Goldberg MJ, Bartoshesky LE. Congenital hand anomaly: etiology and associated malformations. Hand Clin 1985;1(3):405–15.

67. Manske PR. Longitudinal failure of upper limb formation. J Bone Joint Surg Am 1996;78:1600–23.

68. Hirshowitz B, Karev A, Rousso M. Combined double Z-plasty and Y-V advancement for thumb web contracture. Hand 1975;7(3):291–3.

69. Woolf RM, Broadbent TR. The four-flap z-plasty. Plast Reconstr Surg 1972;49:48–51.

70. Miura T, Komada T. Simple method for reconstruction of the cleft hand with an adducted thumb. Plast Reconstr Surg 1979;64(1):65–7.

71. Snow JW, Littler JW. Surgical treatment of cleft hand. In: Sanvenero-Rosselli G, editor. Transactions of the Fourth International Congress of Plastic and Reconstructive Surgery. Edition 1. Rome and Amsterdam: Excerpta Medica Foundation; 1967.

72. Wood VE. The cleft hand (central deficiencies). In: Green DP, editor. Operative hand surgery, edition 1. New York: Churchill Livingstone; 1988.

73. Kay SP, Wiberg M. Toe to hand transfer in children. Part I. Technical aspects. J Hand Surg [Br] 1996;21:723–34.

74. Brown JM, Tickle C. Retinoids and the molecular basis of limb patterning. Comp Biochem Physiol 1992;103A:641–7.

75. Tickle C. Experimental embryology as applied to the upper limb. J Hand Surg [Br] 1987;12(3):294–300.

76. Tickle C, Summerbell D, Wolpert L. Positional signaling and specification of digits in chick limb morphogenesis. Nature 1975;254:199–202.

77. Carroll RE, Bowers WH. Congenital deficiency of the ulna. J Hand Surg [Am] 1977;2(3):169–74.

78. Ogden JA, Watson HK, Bohne W. Ulnar dysmelia. J Bone Joint Surg Am 1976;58(4):467–75.

79. Riordan DC, Mills EH, Alldredge RH. Congenital absence of the ulna. In Proceedings of the American Society for Surgery of the Hand. J Bone Joint Surg Am 1961;43:614.

80. Straub LR. Congenital absence of the ulna. Am J Surg 1965;109:300–5.

81. Broudy AS, Smith RJ. Deformities of the hand and wrist with ulnar deficiency. J Hand Surg [Am] 1979;4(4):304–15.

82. Johnson J, Omer GE Jr. Congenital ulnar deficiency. Natural history and therapeutic implications. Hand Clin 1985;1(3):499–510.

83. Marcus NA, Omer GE Jr. Carpal deviation in congenital ulnar deficiency. J Bone Joint Surg Am 1984;66(7):1003–7.

84. Miller JK, Wenner SM, Kruger LM. Ulnar deficiency. J Hand Surg [Am] 1986;11(6):822–9.

85. Cole RJ, Manske PR. Classification of ulnar deficiency according to the thumb and first web. J Hand Surg [Am] 1997;22:479–88.

86. Ogino T, Kato H. Clinical and experimental studies on ulnar ray deficiency. Handchir Mikrochir Plast Chir 1988;20(6):330–7.

87. Bayne LG. Ulnar club hand (ulnar deficiencies). In: Green DP, editor, Operative hand surgery, edition 1. New York: Churchill Livingstone; 1982. N.

88. Kummel W, editor. Die missbildungen der extremitaeten durch defekt, verwachsung und ueberzahl, edition 1. Cassel Germany: T.G. Fisher; 1895.

89. Swanson AB, Tada K, Yonenobu K. Ulnar ray deficiency: its various manifestations. J Hand Surg [Am] 1984;9(5):658–64.

90. Havenhill TG, Manske PR, Patel A, et al. Type 0 ulnar longitudinal deficiency. J Hand Surg [Am] 2005; 30(6):1288–93.

91. Blauth W. Der hypoplastische daumen. Arch Orthop 1967;62:225–46.

92. Kelikian H. Congenital deformities of the hand and forearm. Philadelphia: Saunders; 1974.

93. Lloyd-Roberts GC. Treatment of defects of the ulna in children by establishing cross-union with the radius. J Bone Joint Surg Br 1973;55(2):327–30.

Failure of Differentiation Part I: Syndactyly

Michael A. Tonkin, MBBS, MD, FRACS, FRCS EdOrth

KEYWORDS

• Syndactyly • Genetics • Classification • Surgery

Syndactyly is one of the two most common congenital hand anomalies, the other being polydactyly. Both have an incidence of about 1 in 2000 births.[1] Traditionally, syndactyly is considered to be simple when skin alone is involved, complex when there is bone connection, complete when the web involvement includes the nail folds, incomplete or partial when the nail folds are not involved but when the web depth is distal to its normal position, and complicated when there are multiple tissue abnormalities—bones, joints, tendons, muscles and neurovascular bundles (Fig. 1). Synpolydactyly and Apert syndrome are two examples of complicated syndactylies.

Syndactyly occurs as an isolated presentation or as part of a syndrome, such as Poland syndrome or one of the acrocephalosyndactyly syndromes, such as Apert syndrome. Tentamy and McKusick[2] have subclassified isolated syndactylies into five groups according to the affected interdigital space or spaces. Syndactyly type I (SD1) is the most common, affecting the long and ring fingers and second and third toes, complete or partial, often but not always bilateral, at times affecting either hands or feet, and occasionally other fingers. It is most commonly of sporadic occurrence, and subsequently autosomal dominant inheritance, but with incomplete penetrance. Syndactyly type II (SD2) is otherwise known as synpolydactyly (SPD), classically with syndactyly between the long and ring fingers and the fourth and fifth toes with duplication within the syndactylous webs. Syndactyly type III (SD3) affects the ring and little fingers in its isolated form, but also occurs at the other end of the spectrum as part of a syndrome, in oculodentodigital syndrome. Syndactyly type IV (SD4) consists of complete syndactyly of all fingers and is rare, as is syndactyly type V (SD5), in which there are metacarpal and metatarsal fusions of commonly the ring and little fingers or the third and fourth toes.

CLASSIFICATION OF CONGENITAL HAND ANOMALIES—WHERE DOES SYNDACTYLY FIT IN?

Under the International Federation of Societies for Surgery of the Hand (IFSSH)/Swanson classification, syndactyly is considered to be a failure of differentiation.[3–5] When skin alone is involved, the failure of separation may reasonably be attributed to a failure in programmed cell death in the particular web. In its complicated forms, however, the process is less clear. Syndactyly accompanies brachydactyly in the condition known as symbrachydactyly, which is classified either as a transverse failure of formation or a hypoplasia. In combination with ipsilateral chest wall anomalies, symbrachydactyly is termed Poland syndrome. The polydactyly of synpolydactyly is classified as a duplication. Central longitudinal deficiency (longitudinal failure of formation) is another condition in which syndactyly occurs regularly and which excites argument in determining the classification group within which it should be included. The elegant clinical and experimental work of Miura,[6] Ogino,[7] and others has demonstrated the association of syndactyly with polydactyly and clefting. The Japanese Society for Surgery of the Hand has suggested the introduction of an additional group within the IFSSH classification, this being abnormal induction of rays, to cater for this association and includes syndactyly within this group.[8]

Department of Hand Surgery and Peripheral Nerve Surgery, Royal North Shore Hospital, University of Sydney, St Leonards, NSW 2065, Sydney, Australia
E-mail address: mtonkin@med.usyd.edu.au

Hand Clin 25 (2009) 171–193
doi:10.1016/j.hcl.2008.12.004
0749-0712/08/$ – see front matter © 2009 Published by Elsevier Inc.

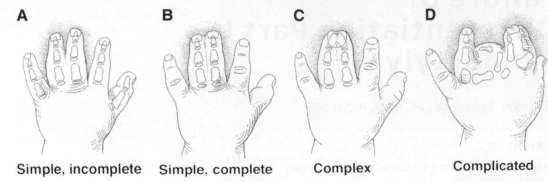

A   **B**   **C**   **D**

Simple, incomplete   Simple, complete   Complex   Complicated

Fig. 1. (*A–D*) Types of syndactyly. (*From* Upton J. Management of disorders of separation—syndactyly. In: Hentz VR, editor. The hand and upper limb (Part 2). In: Mathes SJ, editor. Plastic surgery vol. 8. Philadelphia: Saunders Elsevier; 2006. p. 140; with permission.)

It is apparent that our increasing knowledge of the molecular processes of limb development is modifying our approach to classification of anomalies. The IFSSH/Swanson classification is based on appearance and is unable to satisfactorily incorporate modifications based on the causation of abnormalities at a molecular level. Currently, a descriptive basis for classification probably remains the optimal method to document the anomalies present in any particular limb.[9,10] In the future, classifications based on etiology, site of insult in the developing limb bud, the timing of insult, and abnormalities within molecular pathways may become possible.

EMBRYOLOGY—NORMAL AND ABNORMAL

The limb buds develop as outgrowths in the body wall, the upper limb at 26 to 27 days after fertilization and the lower limb bud at 28 to 30 days. Digits in the upper limb become distinguishable at 41 to 43 days and are fully separated by about 52 to 53 days.[11]

The limb bud consists of a mesenchymal core with overlying ectoderm (**Fig. 2**). The process of growth and differentiation of the limb bud is under complex genetic control. Specialized signal centers control three axes of development.[12] The apical ectodermal ridge (AER) is responsible for controlling proximal-distal outgrowth. Removal of

the AER in experimental models truncates growth.[13] Beneath the apical ectodermal ridge lies the progress zone, in which mesodermal cells are programmed to form specific cell types destined for specific tissues and specific positions within the limb. Control of the anteroposterior or radioulnar axis lies within mesodermal cells within the zone of polarizing activity in the postaxial aspect of the developing limb. Thumb growth is suppressed in this region, allowing development of ulnar digits. Transposition of cells from the zone of polarizing activity to the preaxial or radial aspect of the limb suppresses thumb formation. A mirror hand, or ulnar dimelia, results.[14] The third signal center lies within the cells of the dorsal ectoderm, which control the development of the dorsal-volar characteristics of the limb. Transposition of dorsal ectoderm to the volar aspect of the limb bud results in the dual development of dorsal limb structures.[15] These three signal centers interact through the expression of specific morphogens, which act within cascades of molecular pathways that orchestrate limb development. Fibroblastic growth factors (FGFs) play a major role in the apical ectodermal ridge;[12,13,16,17] sonic hedgehog protein (SHH) in the zone of polarizing activity;[8,12,18] and Wnt-7a is involved in an interaction with the morphogens, Engrailed 1 and Lmx-1b, in determining dorsal and ventral patterning.[15,19–22]

What role do these three axes play in the development of syndactyly? Our knowledge remains imprecise. From day 38, the hand begins to appear in its adult form. Apoptosis is the process of programmed interdigital mesoderm cell death. By 8 weeks, digital separation is almost complete and phalangeal ossification centers are developing.[23] Apoptosis would seem to be mediated by the bone morphogenic protein (BMP) family.[24] These proteins, along with fibroblastic growth factors and members of the homeobox (Hox)

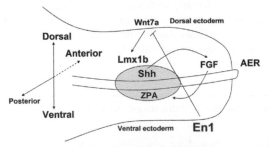

Fig. 2. Diagram of the developing limb bud.

gene family, are expressed in the AER, which seems to be necessary for the induction of cell death. This process is prevented when the AER is removed.[25] BMP-4 is expressed in the interdigital mesenchyme and the joint primordium at the time of distal digit separation. At the end of the embryonic period, when the digits are totally separated, expression of BMP-4 is restricted to the joint-forming region.[26] A decrease in BMP-4 levels leads to a lack of apoptosis in the mesoderm between the fingers and results in syndactyly of the digits. Digit number is related to the width of the limb bud, which in turn depends on the length of the apical ectodermal ridge. A reduction of BMP-4 and altered SHH expression have also been shown to result in polydactyly.[26]

Detailed mechanisms remain unknown but it is becoming clear that a multiplicity of genotypic abnormalities may result in a phenotype in which syndactyly is present. Several clinical presentations that exhibit syndactyly, with or without polydactyly, have a known genetic basis and are worthy of some consideration:

Synpolydactyly

SPD, or SD2, is of autosomal dominant inheritance.[27] The cardinal features are webbing of the middle and ring fingers and the fourth and fifth toes, with partial or complete digital duplications within the syndactylized web. Three genetically distinct malformations are now known—SPD1, SPD2, and SPD3—each with alterations at different chromosome loci. HoxD-13 mutations are responsible for SPD1 features, and FPLN-1 mutations for SPD2 features. In fact, there are several SPD families in which clinical manifestations may present with the typical SPD features, or alternatively with minor variants or unusual phenotypes. Minor variants include simple complete or simple incomplete syndactylies of the third web or simple syndactylies of the second and third toes, as seen in SD1. This finding suggests a variable severity of penetrance rather than isolated syndactyly being a separate condition. Despite this, it is reasonable to limit the term "synpolydactyly" to those presentations that have the following characteristics: involvement of both upper and lower limbs, with the additional digit central in the hands and postaxially in the feet; polydactyly that is accompanied by syndactyly; metacarpal and metatarsal involvement; and complete webbing.

Oculodentodigital Syndrome

Syndactyly of ring and little fingers is accompanied by craniofacial and limb dysmorphism, spastic paraplegia, and neurodegeneration, if completely expressed. Inheritance is autosomal dominant. Mutations in Connexin 43 have been shown to be responsible in oculodentodigital syndrome and in SD3, in which the syndactylies are an isolated finding.[28] Isolated SD3 may be a variant of a syndromic presentation with limited expression.

Greig Cephalopolysyndactyly Syndrome

This condition is caused by an insufficiency of the GLI3 gene, is of autosomal dominant inheritance, and demonstrates typically preaxial or mixed preaxial and postaxial polydactyly, cutaneous syndactyly, ocular hypertelorism, and macrocephaly. A mild presentation may be confused with a nonsyndromic preaxial polysyndactyly. There is also an overlap with other syndromic presentations, which include syndactyly, such as the craniofrontonasal syndrome; the orofacial-digital syndrome, often combining cleft lip and palate, oral abnormalities, and polydactyly and cutaneous syndactyly; and the acro-fronto-cranio-nasal syndrome, which combines preaxial polydactyly and hypertelorism.[29]

Apert Syndrome

Apert syndrome is one of the most common and severe of the craniosynostosis syndromes and is further characterized by midface hypoplasia, syndactyly, and other visceral abnormalities. Most new cases are of sporadic presentation, representing new mutations. Subsequently, inheritance is of an autosomal dominant mode.

The locus has been identified on chromosome 10q26. The abnormal gene has been identified as fibroblastic growth factor receptor 2 (FGFR-2) with one or the other of two specific point mutations, Ser-252 Trp or Pro-253 Arg. Those who have the former mutation present more commonly with cleft palate and the severe craniofacial phenotype. Those who have the latter mutation exhibit a more severe degree of syndactyly.

On occasions polydactyly is present and both preaxial and postaxial polydactyly have been described.

By defining the biomolecular mechanism by which these mutations result in FGFR-2 dysfunction, nonsurgical manipulation of Apert syndrome may be possible in the future.[30,31]

Cleft Hand Complex

This fascinating condition usually affects all four limbs and is of autosomal dominant inheritance. The most common human locus is on chromosome 10. Abnormalities in fibroblastic growth factor 8 (FGF-8) may be causative but this is yet to be proved. In mice, the developmental mechanism underlying the loss of central rays in limbs is dramatic cell death of the apical ectodermal ridge.[32] Ogino and others have recognized the association between clefting, syndactyly, and polydactyly and have created a rat animal model in which cleft hand, central polydactyly, and osseous syndactyly were induced by the same treatment at the same developmental stage. They demonstrate that cleft hand formation proceeds from osseous syndactylies and central polydactylies.[6,7]

It is beyond the scope of this article and the ability of its author to attempt to explain or correlate our current knowledge of the molecular causation of hand anomalies. Nevertheless, it can be seen from the above examples that syndactyly can accompany many presentations, and that already several precise but different genetic abnormalities have been associated with its presence, often in combination with polydactyly and sometimes with clefting. Many pathways may lead to syndactyly. Loss of the integrity of the AER is common to most of these.

SURGICAL TECHNIQUES

When syndactyly is present, there is a relative lack of skin. It is helpful to demonstrate this to parents by simply measuring the circumference of mom or dad's middle and ring fingers separately and comparing their combined measurement with the measurement of the circumference of the two fingers when held together. On average, there is a 30% skin shortage (**Fig. 3**). The elasticity of skin and the ability to transfer skin from areas of relative excess to areas of relative lack may allow cover of the separated digits. Additional skin, mainly through skin grafting but also through the use of regional or distant flaps, is often necessary.

Three components of the digit require reconstruction: the web, the digital skin, and the nail folds when the syndactyly is complete. The many variations of flap design are well illustrated by Upton.[23] The following techniques represent my preferences and the principles on which these preferences are based.

The Web

The characteristics of a normal interdigital web are its relative depth, its hourglass shape, and its proximal to distal, dorsal to palmar inclination of 40 to 45 degrees (**Fig. 4**).[23] There are many variations of web flap design, but most are based on the transposition of a dorsal rectangular flap, a palmar rectangular flap, or interdigitating V-flaps. Many favor the first of these for the reason that, theoretically, a dorsally based rectangular flap, however

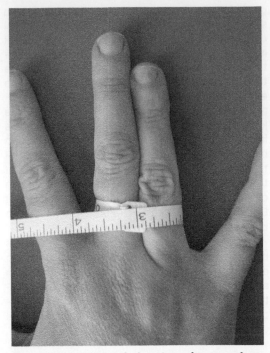

Fig. 3. Measurement of the circumference of two fingers when held together reveals a 30% skin shortage when compared with the skin cover necessary to resurface both digits individually.

modified, best returns the optimal inclination of the web. My own experience is that it is difficult to determine a difference in web inclination at long-term follow-up between those cases in which a dorsal rectangular flap was used and those in which interdigitating V-flaps were used (**Fig. 5**). This inclination may be returned by the mechanical

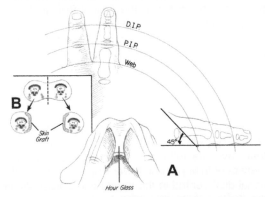

Fig. 4. Characteristics of the web space. (A) Relative web depth, dorsal to palmar inclination and hourglass shape of the interdigital web. (B) Indication of a relative skin deficiency. (From Upton J. Management of disorders of separation—syndactyly. In: Hentz VR, editor. The hand and upper limb (Part 2). In: Mathes SJ, editor. Plastic surgery vol. 8. Philadelphia: Saunders Elsevier; 2006. p. 140; with permission.)

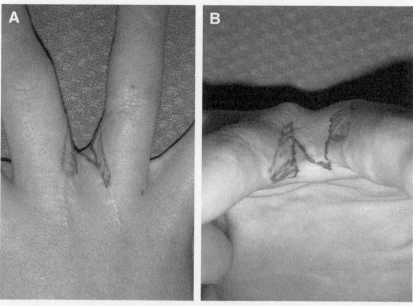

Fig. 5. (*A, B*) Reformation of dorsal to palmar interdigital web inclination following reconstruction with interdigitating v-flaps. Note the advancement of the palmar flap to the side of the dorsal flap rather than to its base.

web stresses in normal hand activity rather than the design of the flap itself, although scar contraction may alter the contour, whatever design is used.

In a simple syndactyly of one web space, it is relatively easy to identify the appropriate depth of the web on the palmar side. The second and

third web spaces lie at the same level and the fourth web space proximal to this. It is my practice to place the reconstructed web at a depth just proximal to its normal web level, perhaps by 1 or 2 mm, allowing for some creep (**Fig. 6**). If using a dorsal flap, this should extend two thirds of the

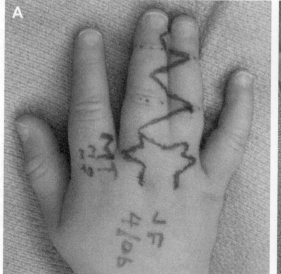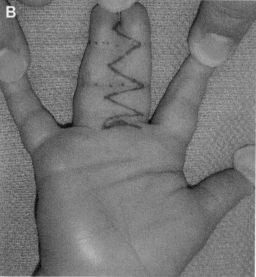

Fig. 6. (*A, B*) Design of dorsal flap; position of palmar web depth 2 mm proximal to normal level; elevation of interdigital flaps extending to midline of each digit. Transverse lines drawn around the digits indicate the levels of interdigitation of palmar and dorsal flaps. Note the concavity at the distal end of the dorsal flap, which matches the convexity of the palmar incision at the base of the fingers, which allows a more proximal inset of the dorsal web flap at its margins. This placement is designed to diminish the possibility of web creep. The triangular extensions onto the dorsum of each digit just distal to metacarpophalangeal joints allow rotation of this skin from a redundant area through 90° to the dorsolateral aspects of the digits where skin is deficient.

length of a line drawn from midpoint of metacarpal heads to midpoint of proximal interphalangeal joints (**Figs. 6** and **7**). It is more difficult to determine the correct web depth in cases of multiple syndactylies and in complicated syndactylies with multiple bone abnormalities. Normal webs lie roughly halfway between the proximal interphalangeal joint crease and the distal palmar crease; this can be a useful basis for placement of the palmar skin incision. The ability to achieve this depth may be controlled by other anatomic anomalies, however, such as distal neurovascular bifurcation, distal tendon bifurcation, and anomalies within the skeleton. In such cases interdigitating V-flaps are more forgiving in that the length of overlap of the flaps may be varied according to need. The tip of one flap need not be sutured to the base of the other; rather the tip of one may be sutured to the side of the other as appropriate (see **Fig. 5**). Distal bifurcation of the artery may prevent proximal web placement. It may be necessary to tie off one digital artery if a distal bifurcation prevents the surgeon from creating an adequate web depth. An intraneural dissection of the common digital nerve usually overcomes a restriction created by distal nerve bifurcation. Awareness of the vascular anatomy on the other side of the digit is necessary, particularly in multiple and complicated syndactylies. It is dangerous to operate on both sides of the same digit simultaneously. In staged procedures, the surgeon should make certain that one proper digital artery is retained with each digit.

Digital Flaps

For mobile digits, zig-zag incisions are necessary so that scar contraction across flexion creases does not result in deformity. Some favor acutely angled flaps in which there may be a slightly increased risk for flap tip necrosis. Others favor more obtusely angled flaps. The more obtuse the angle, the more likely is the scar to develop a straight line with growth, leading to flexion contractures or angulatory deformity. Regardless, the principle should be to raise the flap to the midline of each digit (see **Fig. 6**). Careful planning is necessary such that, when inset, the flaps interdigitate. Some plan flap elevation such that one digit becomes the dominant digit, receiving full or near-full local skin cover, leaving gaps on the adjacent digit for skin grafting. I prefer an equal distribution of skin to each digit. It is not necessary to place a needle through the web to ensure that dorsal and palmar incisions are placed at the correct level. Transverse lines drawn around the digits are satisfactory (see **Fig. 6**). Those concerned about correct flap orientation for each digit place an arrow pointing toward the tip of each flap. At each level, the arrows must point in the same direction during rotation of the digit complex.

During flap elevation judicious defatting is undertaken, while being careful to preserve vessels and skin viability. Interdigital fat is excised around both neurovascular bundles, which are identified distally and dissected proximally. For simple syndactylies, the bifurcation of the artery determines the depth of proximal dissection.

The natatory fascia should be removed from the web as should the fascia of the lateral digital sheet along each side of the digit. The retention of tight fascia in continuity may lead to deformity with growth. The flap design should be planned such that there is no continuity between the incision at the base of the web and the incision at the base of each digit, because this continuity may lead to web creep with growth, more so if scar contraction is significant (**Fig. 8**).

Nail Folds

In complete syndactylies, particularly when the nails are joined, a satisfactory recreation of nail folds along the contiguous borders of the digits is necessary for an optimal appearance and avoidance of nail-nail bed irritation. Skin and pulp are required. The transposition flaps described by Buck-Gramcko are ideal (**Fig. 9**).[33] These flaps should be raised before the terminal parts of the digit are separated, because a slip of the knife may transect the mid-aspect of the nail fold flap to be raised.

Alternative methods include the attachment of a thenar flap at the time of a preliminary distal digit separation, with completion of separation performed at the time of division and insetting of the flap.[34,35] Free toe pulp flaps are another

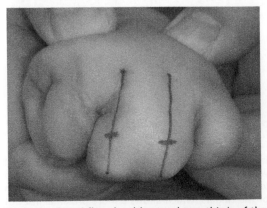

Fig. 7. The dorsal flap should extend two thirds of the length of a line drawn from the dimples of the metacarpal heads to the proximal interphalangeal joints.

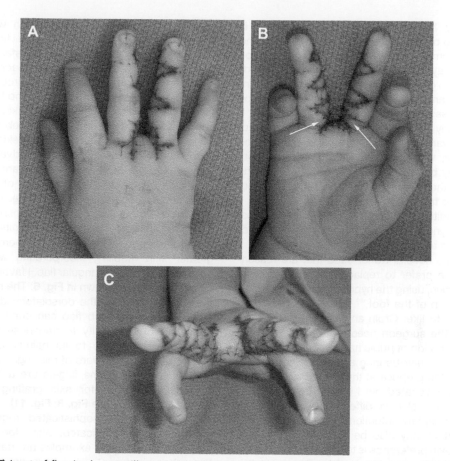

Fig. 8. (*A–C*) Inset of flap in the case illustrated in **Fig. 6**. Transverse closure of the defect from which the dorsal triangular flaps are elevated is possible. No skin grafts were used. The arrows point to the bases of the palmar flaps of each digit with no continuity of scar between the base of the dorsal web flap and the palmar side of each finger. Complete cover without skin grafting is possible in most cases of simple complete syndactyly. The interdigital webspace is broad and of satisfactory depth.

possibility.[36,37] Full-thickness grafts do not provide adequate bulk but can be taken with several millimeters of fat. Consideration needs to be given to appropriate soft tissue cover of exposed distal interphalangeal joints when there is a complex syndactyly with bony connection along the substance of the distal phalanx.[37]

Skin Cover

There is a relative lack of skin. Recently there has been a move toward avoiding skin grafts.[38–40] I believe that it is possible to avoid skin grafts in many instances but that one should not be a slave to this principle. In many instances of simple

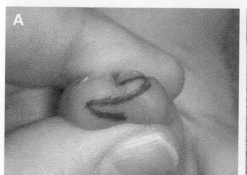

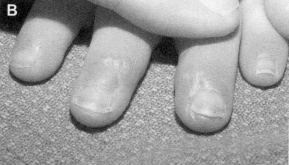

Fig. 9. (*A, B*) Buck-Gramcko nail fold flaps with satisfactory postoperative result.

syndactyly, both complete and incomplete, it is possible to obtain skin cover without grafting and without compromising the result. The surgeon should always ask him or herself whether avoidance of skin grafting compromises the web reconstruction and whether tight suture of flaps compromises flap viability or that of the digits. If there is any doubt, skin grafts should be used. The disadvantages are only those of the duration of surgery, which is unimportant; pigmentation, which may be less than ideal, particularly in the hands of those from black races; and failure of the graft to take, which is a problem.

The addition of skin is necessary in most complex syndactylies and in complicated syndactylies, such as those of Apert syndrome.

There are several donor sites that are reasonable. Some prefer to replace glabrous skin with glabrous skin, using the hypothenar eminence[41–43] or the instep of the foot,[44] perhaps not glabrous but closer to like. Groin and abdominal skin are popular. The surgeon needs to be aware of the likely distribution of pubic hair because skin transferred from a hair-bearing area will produce hair. Skin from the prepuce at the time of circumcision has been advocated but I do not favor this. The quality of the skin is different, pigmentation is significant, and the infection risk is increased.[45,46] Pigmentation may also be a concern with groin skin. My own preference is to use skin from the antecubital fossa, as advocated by Benatar.[47] It is appropriate for those occasions when skin grafting is necessary but large amounts of skin are not required. The donor site is based at the elbow flexion crease, with the transverse scar healing nicely within the crease (**Fig. 10**).

I have not discussed the advantages and disadvantages of full-thickness skin grafting and split-thickness skin grafting. In my opinion, the latter is to be condemned. Skin contraction within the growing digit is unsatisfactory and the quality and robustness of split skin is unsatisfactory.

Necessity for addition of skin is decreased by judicious defatting to decrease the circumference of each digit, loose suture of flaps, and transposition of skin from areas of redundant skin to places lacking skin. The configuration of web flaps has been modified in an attempt to avoid skin grafting. A dorsal island pedicle flap may be advanced and rotated into the web.[48–50] The disadvantage is the extension of scar to the dorsal part of the hand such that the scars are more visible. Niranjan[38] and Giele[51] have advocated the transposition of skin from the dorsal aspect of the digits, distal to the metacarpophalangeal joints, where there is greater skin mobility, incorporating wings into a standard dorsal rectangular flap. I favor a modification of these as shown in **Fig. 6**. The rotation of dorsal skin to cover the dorsolateral defects on either side of the web flap can compromise to some extent the ability to transpose the distal end of the web flap to its palmar base. The surgeon should be aware of this. Again, scars on the dorsal areas of the fingers are a little more obvious. The need for skin grafting may be avoided, however (see **Fig. 8; Fig. 11**).

Unusually, more sophisticated regional and distant flaps are indicated, often for first web reconstruction. Some examples are described in the subsequent sections. I have no experience with tissue expansion to provide for the relative skin shortage of syndactyly. The high incidence of complications seems to negate the benefits.[52]

Incomplete Syndactyly

When the incomplete syndactyly extends to a length equal to or beyond two thirds of the

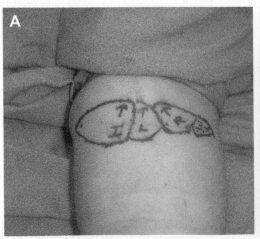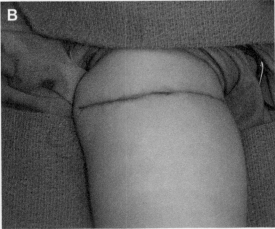

Fig. 10. (*A, B*) Use of the cubital fossa crease for digit skin grafting.

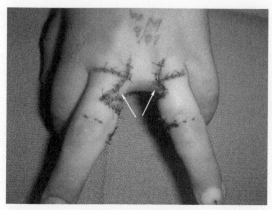

Fig. 11. Inset of wings (*arrowed*) following rotation through 90° without skin grafting.

distance between metacarpophalangeal and proximal interphalangeal joints, I favor a formal dorsally based rectangular flap, as for complete syndactylies. When the webbing is proximal to this, however, one of many variations of local flaps is appropriate. A modification of the double reverse Z-plasty works nicely (**Fig. 12**).[53] Rectangular flaps, among many others, are another option.[23]

The First Web

Release of the syndactylized thumb is a surgical procedure that provides significant functional benefit. Different techniques are applicable to mild, moderate, and severe first web space deficiencies. For mild deficiency, I prefer a four-flap web plasty, which provides good contour (**Fig. 13**). A simple Z-plasty tends to create a V shape.[54,55] As for incomplete digital syndactylies, there are multiple flap designs that are appropriate.[23]

For cases of moderate restriction of the first web space, more tissue may need to be brought to the web. Many forms of transposition, rotation, or

rotation-advancement flaps have been described.[53,56–66] Skin grafting is often necessary. Upton[23] has pointed out that it is better to graft along the lateral border of thumb or index finger, and not directly across the webspace, nor on the dorsal aspects of thumb or index finger. Buck-Gramcko's dorsal advancement flap is effective (**Fig. 14**).

For severe cases, such as in Apert syndrome, some symbrachydactylies, a mitten hand, or for first web syndactyly in combination with clefting, regional or distant tissue may be necessary. Sometimes, removal of one digit provides extra skin. The placement of dorsal incisions for the first web space must be carefully considered if these compromise the subsequent elevation of dorsal flaps for separation of the digits. Regional pedicle flaps can be of benefit but entail an assessment of donor site morbidity. A radial forearm flap or a posterior interosseous artery flap are two that are more commonly used (**Fig. 15**).[67–70] The latter has the disadvantage of introducing hair-bearing skin to the first web. Distant pedicle flaps, such as the groin flap, are rarely indicated. On occasion, free vascularized tissue transfer may be used. Free groin or lateral arm flaps are two examples.[71,72]

In moderate and severe cases, the fascia of the first dorsal interosseous and adductor pollicis should be released. Anatomic variations of the princeps pollicis artery are common. The surgeon should be aware of this and ensure that its integrity is maintained. Release or excision of anomalous muscles and release of the carpometacarpal joint are sometimes necessary. Wire fixation to maintain the web width during healing is appropriate.

Suture Material

Inert suture material probably decreases the inflammatory response to foreign material. Some prefer the use of fine monofilament sutures, such as 6-0 Prolene. These require removal. The number of sutures and the age of the child are such that a second general anesthetic, at 2 to 3 weeks after digital separation, is necessary. Others use absorbable sutures at the risk of a greater inflammatory response. My own observation is that at 6 months after surgery there is little difference between the two, even if there is an increased inflammatory response initially with the absorbable suture. I use 6-0 Vicryl Rapide. It is relatively fine and dissolves or rubs out following bathing or massage at about 4 weeks after surgery. For those cases in which the surgeon is aware of an increased risk of hypertrophic scar formation, and in surgery of revision of excessive scarring, it is not unreasonable to

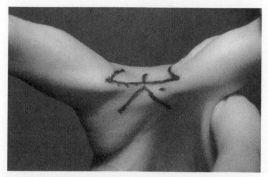

Fig. 12. Double reverse Z-plasty with modification for mild simple incomplete syndactylies.

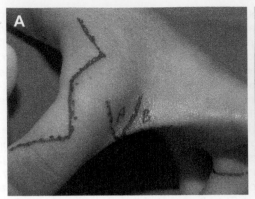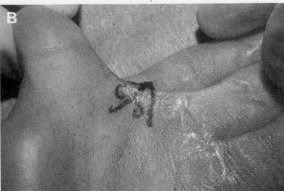

Fig. 13. (*A, B*) The four-flap web plasty for mild first web syndactyly.

add the insult of a second anesthetic for removal of sutures, particularly if one is dealing with syndactyly release when there is overgrowth of digits. The incidence of keloid formation is significantly increased and one should use every possible method available to decrease that risk.[73,74]

Dressings

I use Vaseline gauze and strips of moistened, well–wrung out thin wool placed longitudinally and obliquely, not circumferentially (**Fig. 16**). Chloromycetin ointment is beneficial in application of the gauze to the contour of the digit, and may decrease the risk of infection. The dressings are

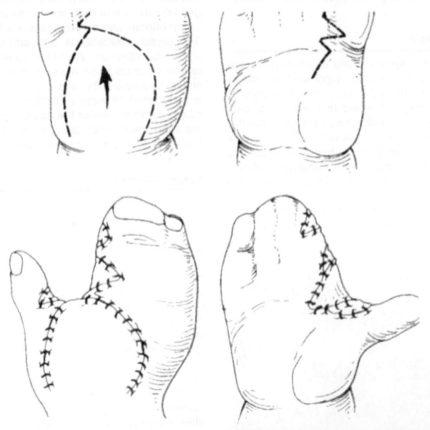

Fig. 14. Buck-Gramcko first web plasty. (*From* Upton J. Management of disorders of separation—syndactyly. In: Hentz VR, editor. The hand and upper limb (Part 2). In: Mathes SJ, editor. Plastic surgery vol. 8. Philadelphia: Saunders Elsevier; 2006. p. 158; with permission.)

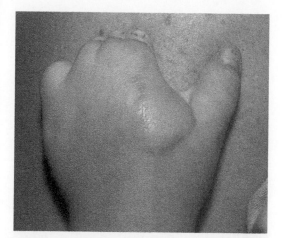

Fig. 15. A case of symbrachydactyly in which a posterior interosseous artery flap was used for a moderate to severe first web syndactyly, leaving dorsal skin available for future digital separation.

then built up with layers of thin wool so that there is an even pressure within the web and along the adjacent sides of digits. It is particularly important when skin grafts have been used to apply a gentle compressive pressure to prevent shearing, without interfering with blood flow within the relatively denuded digital arteries and with venous drainage. The final picture is one of dressings closely applied, but not under tension, within the digital interspaces, developed to a boxing glove appearance, with or without simple plaster slabs. The dressing is retained by placing 3-in U-shaped Elastoplast stirrups around the elbow to prevent proximal migration of the dressing or complete dissociation of the dressing from the patient (**Fig. 17**).

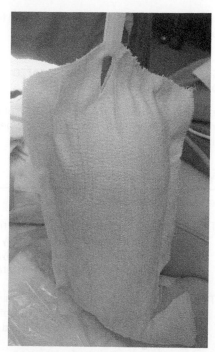

Fig. 17. Dressings with thin plaster slabs secured by 3-in Elastoplast.

Some change the dressings at 1 week. I prefer to leave them for 2 or sometimes 3 weeks when there has been extensive skin grafting. The dressings are then changed in the clinic. If there is any moisture, moist dressings are used until healing is obtained. The use of Coban compressive wrapping of the digits is routine to provide an even pressure over the healing scars. If scarring seems to be excessive, further wound therapy, such as the use of silicon, is indicated.

Timing of Surgery

Simple, complete syndactylies are released at about 12 to 15 months. Long-term results are not compromised by waiting longer, however.

Fourth web syndactyly, particularly if complex, may lead to angulatory and rotatory deformities at interphalangeal joins and are better released earlier. The first web should be freed at 6 months or thereabouts.

In some complicated cases, the small size of phalanges and the presence of difficult-to-define skeletal anatomy may prevent optimal surgery. The surgeon must decide whether to release and attend to digit deformity secondarily, or alternatively whether to delay and attend to all components of the syndactyly simultaneously when satisfied that an error of excision or technique will not compromise digit alignment and growth,

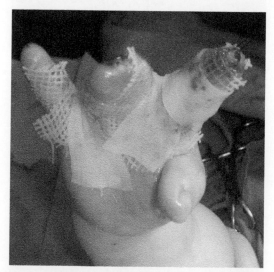

Fig. 16. Application of Vaseline gauze and strips of moist wool secured with Chloromycetin ointment.

or joint stability and motion. Such cases need to be assessed individually. If in doubt, wait.

SURGICAL TECHNIQUES FOR COMPLICATED SYNDACTYLIES

The principles remain the same. It is useful to describe some techniques applicable to specific conditions.

Apert Syndrome

These hands are divided into three types:

> Type 1: The index, middle, and ring fingers are joined by a complex distal syndactyly and the little finger by a simple syndactyly; the thumb is free but deviated in the radial plane (**Fig. 18**).
>
> Type 2: The thumb is included in a simple syndactyly and there is splaying of the central metacarpals of the long and ring fingers (**Fig. 19**).
>
> Type 3: The skeletal union is of all digits and is often complicated; radial deviation of the thumb may not be present (**Fig. 20**).

In all there is symphalangism of the interphalangeal joints of the central three digits and of the proximal interphalangeal joint of the little finger. There is commonly a four–five metacarpal synostosis, which limits optimal motion of the otherwise more mobile little finger.

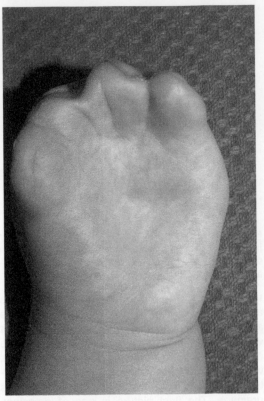

Fig. 19. Type 2 Apert hand.

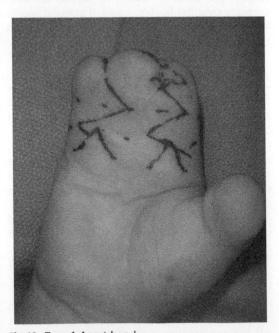

Fig. 18. Type 1 Apert hand.

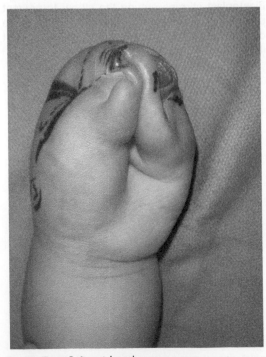

Fig. 20. Type 3 Apert hand.

Interdigitating V-flaps for web reconstruction allow the surgeon some freedom in obtaining a pleasing level of web depth (**Fig. 21**). Some prefer a dorsal rectangular flap in the second web. Web creep is not uncommon and may be related to a relative increase in index finger ray growth. The rectangular flap is more easily advanced during revision surgery.[23] Because the digits are immobile, straight line incisions with grafting are satisfactory for digital cover (see **Fig. 21**). Habenicht[75] uses lateral digital distraction to separate the rays, gaining extra skin by this process. Distal bony corrections are divided at the time of application of the distractor. Buck-Gramcko nail fold reconstruction usually provides satisfactory nail folds.

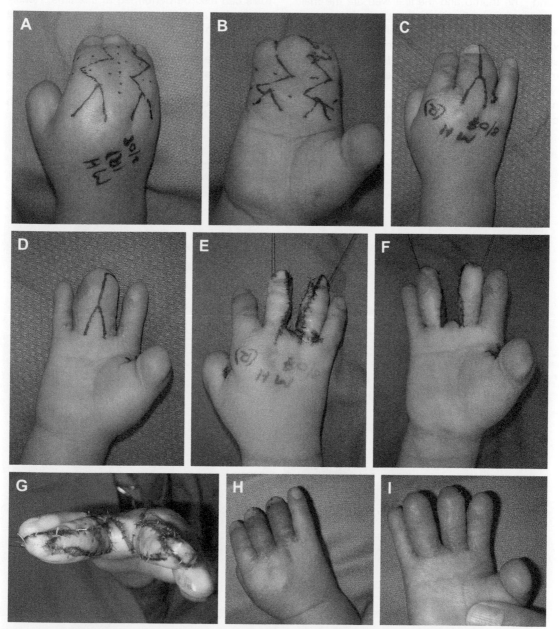

Fig. 21. (A, B) Apert hand at the time of simultaneous bilateral 2nd and 4th web release. Note the interdigitating v-flaps for the webs, which allow some freedom in placement of the web depth. (C, D) Longitudinal incision used in 2nd stage release of the third webs. (E–G) Digital cover requires skin grafting regardless of whether zig-zag flaps are raised on palmar palmar (A) and dorsal (B) sides of the digits, or whether longitudinal incisions are used (C, D). (H, I) Early postoperative results are shown.

It is my practice to perform bilateral simultaneous procedures to decrease the number of operations. In type 1 hands, the second and fourth webs are released at the first stage and the third web at the second stage (see **Fig. 21**). In type 2 hands, the first and third webs are released initially followed by the second and fourth. In type 3 hands, a decision needs to be made as to whether it is more appropriate to aim for a three-fingered hand. The thumb and the first web are the main components of function. Removal of the index finger ray in combination with release of the fourth web, followed by release of the third web in the second stage, provides optimal function and, for most eyes, a satisfactory appearance (**Fig. 22**). Neither the three-fingered nor the four-fingered hand will have normal appearance. This decision can only be made in consultation with parents.

Photographs and models of surgical results are helpful in this discussion.

The angulated thumb is dealt with in a third procedure, perhaps between 4 and 6 years of age. There may be need for extra skin across the concavity of the deformity, in conjunction with a proximal phalanx osteotomy and, at times, in combination with lengthening.[23]

The release of the four–five metacarpal synostosis can also be performed at this time. Recurrence is a problem, however, and some interposition material is appropriate. It is possible to elevate a subcutaneous fat graft to interpose between the bases of the fourth and fifth metacarpals. Others have advised interposition of a free fascial graft or hydrated cadaveric fascia lata, wrapped circumferentially around the fifth metacarpal.[23]

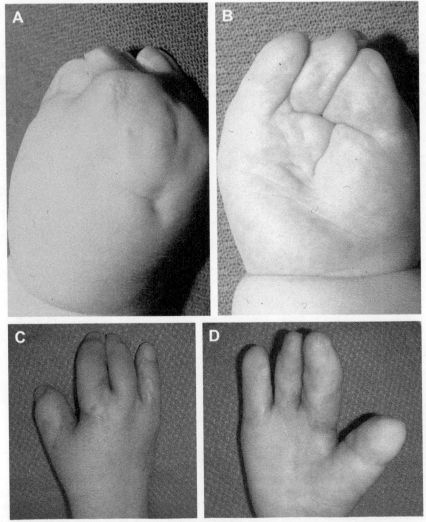

Fig. 22. (A–D) Type 3 Apert hand and surgical result following removal of the index finger ray.

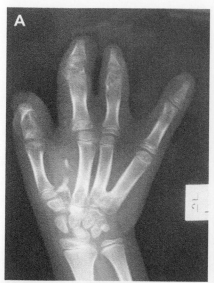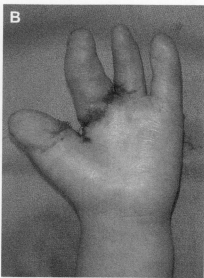

Fig. 23. (*A*) Radiograph of abducted little finger with four–five metacarpal synostosis before surgery to revise first and second webs and correct alignment of little finger. (*B*) Postoperative result.

The timing of surgery depends on the timing of craniofacial surgery and any other procedures that may take priority. If nail fold infection intervenes, this should be attended to before formal digital release. It may be preferable to release the thumb in type 3 hands by the age of 6 months or thereabouts. If the thumb is free or held by skin alone, the aim is to complete all digital separations by the age of 18 months. Revision surgery to webs is performed as necessary, with realignment osteotomies at the age of 8 to 10 years (**Fig. 23**).

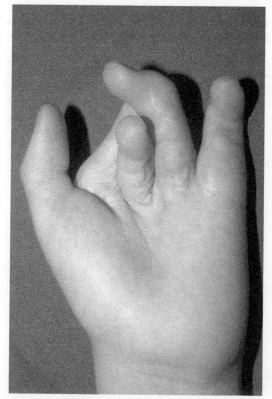

Fig. 24. Ill-advised separation in a case of symbrachydactyly, with resultant instability and deviation.

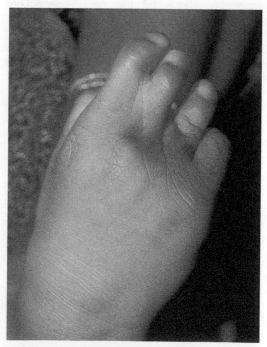

Fig. 25. Symbrachydactyly with unstable digits stabilized by skin bridges. Aggressive release is inadvisable.

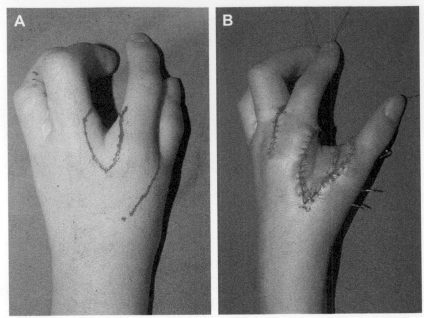

Fig. 26. (*A, B*) Dorsal view of a Snow-Littler transposition from the cleft to the first web with a palmar based flap.

Symbrachydactyly

Symbrachydactyly, short finger type, presents some specific problems because of the lack of digit length and underdevelopment of all digital structures. The surgeon should be wary of joint instability following separation of digits rendered reasonably stable by their skin connections (**Fig. 24**).

Each joint of all fingers to be separated should be assessed individually. One helpful indicator of metacarpophalangeal joint instability is the presence of dimpling in combination with excessive palmar displacement of the proximal phalanx on the metacarpal head (**Fig. 25**).

Apparent digit length may be increased by a more proximal web placement, with or without transverse metacarpal ligament division.

Multiple Syndactylies

The unilateral mitten hand presents similar problems to those faced in the management of Apert hands. The skeletal elements of central rays are

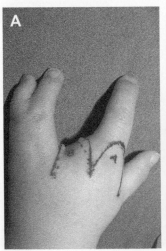
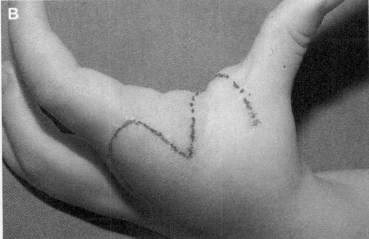

Fig. 27. (*A, B*) Pre- and postoperative views demonstrating the use of a dorsally based bilobed flap to close the cleft and provide skin for the first web.

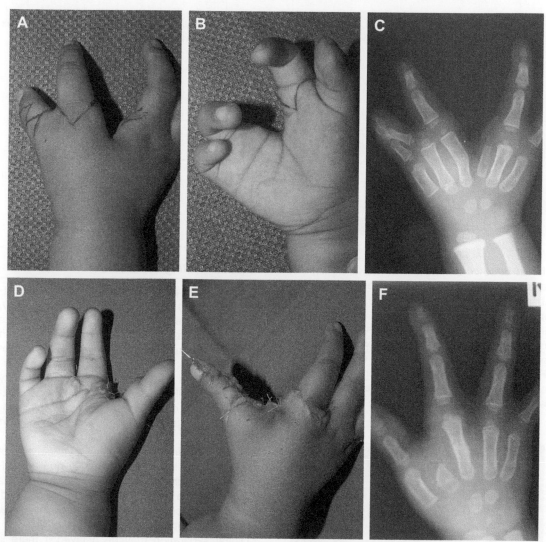

Fig. 28. Corrective osteotomy of middle finger with excision of extra metacarpal within cleft. (*A, B*) Excision of index finger, which was involved in a complex syndactyly with the thumb. (*C*) Radiograph showing a cleft hand and syndactyly of the thumb. (*D, E*) Draping of the skin from the cleft into the first web incisions. (*F*) Radiograph of early postoperative results.

often deficient and, at times, digit excision is indicated. Dorsal skin may be required for digital webs, limiting the usefulness of a dorsal rotation advancement flap for the first web. In these instances, regional and distant flaps may be used as previously described (see **Fig. 15**).

Central Longitudinal Deficiency (Cleft Hand)

The usual principles apply. Several techniques nicely transfer excess skin from the cleft to a syndactylized first web. Although the Snow-Littler transposition flap has fallen out of favor, I find it useful (**Figs. 26** and **27**).[76] Upton prefers a simpler approach in which a circumferential incision of the index finger to be transposed ulnarward is

combined with straight-line incisions in the first web and a Barsky-type flap in the cleft.[77] Following transposition, the skin is simply draped into the first web and the flaps are then contoured as required, with or without a Z-plasty. Release of the thumb adductor and the first dorsal interosseous from the first metacarpal allows satisfactory index finger transposition (**Fig. 28**).

Central Polysyndactyly

These hands present specific difficulties and the outcomes are often less than satisfactory. Management of skin is not the problem. Rather, the surgeon must decide which parts of which rays should be removed. I believe that the principle

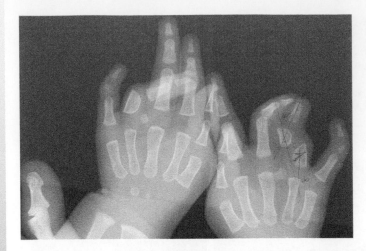

Fig. 29. Preoperative planning for skeletal realignment in a case of complex central polysyndactyly.

should be to compromise on the side of stiffness rather than instability, the latter resulting from an absence of stabilizing soft tissues or underdeveloped, intrinsically unstable joints. Rotational and angular deformities are often complex. It is ideal to attempt to realign the skeleton and stabilize joints, when needed, at the time of digit separation (**Fig. 29**). Future growth commonly alters what initially may have appeared to be a satisfactory result.

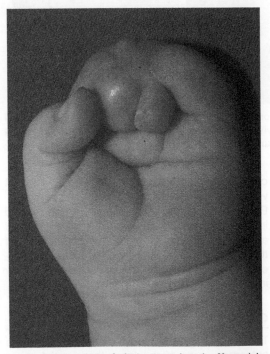

Fig. 30. Confluence of digits in a hand affected by constriction ring syndrome. Note the connection of the little finger to the middle and index digits, forming a connection over the dorsum of the ring finger.

Constriction Ring Syndrome

Release of the acrosyndactyly of multiple shortened digits can be gratifying for patient, family, and surgeon. Separation of a confluence of digits often provides significant improvements in appearance and function. Although there are not usually bony connections, the digits may be intertwined and it is necessary to determine clinically and radiologically the continuity of distal and proximal parts of all digits (**Fig. 30**). At times, it is inappropriate to separate a confluence of two short digits.

The skin circling the cleft of acrosyndactyly is of little benefit, being thin and of poor quality. Full-thickness skin grafting is beneficial. Terminal parts of bones at the level of amputation are tapered. Formal pulp reconstruction is superior to a distal adherent scar at the tip of these digits.

Digital separation may be delayed if there is a concern about distal vascularity. Staged procedures assist in avoiding tissue loss. Scar at the level of the insult may be better removed initially, with flap advancement, before secondary digit separation.[78]

Complications

Complications are a consequence of flap necrosis, infection, skin graft loss, and scar contraction. In complex and complicated syndactylies, joint instability and angulatory and rotational deformities are more common.[41,46,60,79–102] The principles espoused in this article assist in diminishing the incidence of these complications. When encountered, small areas of skin loss can be treated with dressings. Any substantial area of skin necrosis or failure of skin graft should be treated by excision and revision grafting, because healing by secondary intention is likely to lead to scar contraction. Once scar contractures have developed, the appropriate treatment is excision, with advancement of flaps where possible in web spaces and liberal use of skin grafting in the digits. Bony deformity is best treated by osteotomy but, in these instances, we are trying to catch up with problems that are better avoided by meticulous planning at the time of initial intervention. Soft tissue reconstruction of joint instability is difficult. Fusion may be necessary.

One interesting angulatory deformity is that occurring at the distal interphalangeal joints following separation of a complex syndactyly. The deviations may be convergent or divergent and the direction is not always predictable preoperatively. A K-wire across the distal interphalangeal joint at the time of separation, in combination with the use of local tissue to reconstruct collateral ligaments, assists in diminishing the degree of deformity.

Web creep is not uncommon (**Fig. 31**), but if the surgeon plans appropriately, avoids continuity of scar between web and digit, plans flaps to avoid deformity with scar contraction and growth, removes distorting fascia, and attends to areas of delayed healing appropriately, this complication incidence can be decreased. The surgeon does not have absolute control over the formation of hypertrophic scar, nor of keloid scar. In the presence of the former, the scar should be allowed to mature and should be treated aggressively with physical measures. If deformity is intervening, excision and grafting must be performed early. Keloid in the hand is uncommon but the risk is greatly increased when syndactyly is accompanied by digit overgrowth (**Fig. 32**). In these instances, the prophylactic use of methotrexate has been shown to be of benefit and has also been shown to suppress the recurrence of keloid when used at the time of revision surgery.[73,74] This result remains a complication for all surgeons to fear. It is more common when operating on syndactyly of the foot accompanied by digital overgrowth, and when these conditions coexist the surgeon should be wary and the parents of the patient should be warned.

Separation of syndactyly is a satisfactory procedure but not one without complications. When the indication is for appearance alone, such as in the simple complete or incomplete syndactyly of the second web space of the foot, scarring

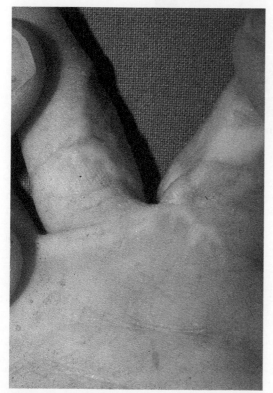

Fig. 31. Mild to moderate web creep demonstrating connection of scar between the web flap base and the palmar aspect of the digits.

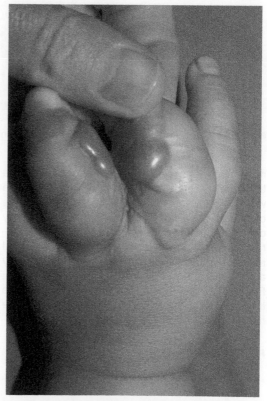

Fig. 32. Keloid formation following separation of a simple syndactyly of the third web space between digits with overgrowth.

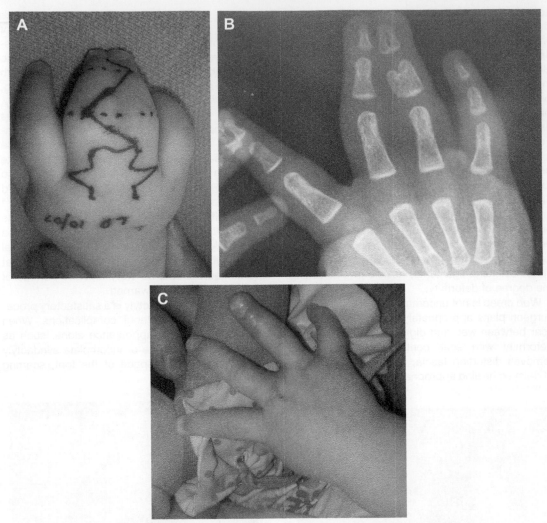

Fig. 33. (*A–C*) Satisfactory clinical appearance following syndactyly release for a complicated syndactyly.

may result in a significantly poorer appearance than that present preoperatively. Drawing a line with a black pen, which simulates the appearance of a cleft to all but the most acute eye, may convince a parent or teenager to consider a temporary or permanent tattoo rather than surgical release. Photographs of our worst results may assist parents and patients in decision making. Few would deny, however, that surgical release is indicated in most cases of syndactyly in the hand (**Fig. 33**).

REFERENCES

1. Flatt A. The care of congenital hand anomalies. St. Louis (MO): CV Mosby; 1977. p. 99–117, 228–48.
2. Tentamy SA, McKusick VA. The genetics of hand malformations. New York: The National Foundation March of Dimes; 1978.
3. Swanson AB. A classification for congenital limb malformations. J Hand Surg 1976;1:8–22.
4. Swanson AB, Swanson GD, Tada K. A classification for congenital limb malformation. J Hand Surg 1983;8:693–702.
5. Knight SL, Kay SPJ. Classification of congenital anomalies. In: Gupta A, Kay SPJ, Scheker LR, editors. The growing hand. London: Harcourt; 2000. p. 125–35.
6. Miura T. Syndactyly and split hand. Hand 1976;8:125–30.
7. Ogino T. Teratogenic relationship between polydactyly, syndactyly and cleft hand. J Hand Surg 1990;15:201–9.
8. Riddle RD, Tabin CJ. How limbs develop. Sci Am 1999;280:74–7.
9. Tonkin MA. Description of congenital hand anomalies: a personal view. J Hand Surg 2006;31B:489–97.

10. Tonkin MA. Classification des anomalies congenitales de al main [Classification of congenital hand anomalies.] Chirurgie de la main. 2008;27SI: S27–34 [in French].

11. Moore KL. The developing human. Philadelphia: Saunders; 1982.

12. Tickle C. Molecular basis of limb development. Biochem Soc Trans 1994;22:565–9.

13. Niswander L, Tickle C, Vogel A, et al. FGF-4 replaces the apical ectodermal ridge and directs outgrowth and patterning of the limb. Cell 1993; 75:579–87.

14. Tickle C. Genetics and limb development. Dev Genet 1996;19:1–8.

15. Johnson RL, Tabin C. Molecular models for vertebrate limb development. Cell 1997;90:979–90.

16. Vogel A, Rodriguez C, Izpisua-Belmonte JC. Involvement of FGF-8 in initiation, outgrowth and patterning of the vertebrate limb. Development 1996;122:1737–50.

17. Niswander L, Martin GR. FGF-4 expression during gastrulation myogenesis, limb and tooth development in the mouse. Development 1992;114:755–68.

18. Riddle RD, Johnson RL, Laufer B, et al. Sonic hedgehog mediates the polarizing activity of the ZPA. Cell 1993;75:1401–16.

19. Parr BA, McMahon AP. Dorsalizing signal Wnt-7a required for normal polarity of D-V and A-P axes of mouse limb. Nature 1995;374:350–3.

20. Chen H, Lun Y, Ovchinnikov D, et al. Limb and kidney defects in Lmx 1b mutant mice suggest an involvement of LMX1B in human nail-patella syndrome. Nat Genet 1998;19:51–5.

21. Dreyer SD, Zhou G, Baldini A, et al. Mutations in LMX1B cause abnormal skeletal patterning and renal dysplasia in nail-patella syndrome. Nat Genet 1998;19:47–50.

22. Riddle RD, Ensini M, Nelson C, et al. Induction of the LIM homeobox gene Lmx1 by WNT7a establishes dorso-ventral pattern in the vertebrate limb. Cell 1995;83:631–40.

23. Upton J. Management of disorders of separation—syndactyly. In: Hentz VR, editor. The hand and upper limb (Part 2). In: Mathes SJ, editor. Plastic surgery, Vol 8. Philadelphia: Saunders Elsevier; 2006. p. 139–84.

24. Clarkson P. Poland's syndactyly. Guys Hosp Rep 1962;111:335–46.

25. Ellis HM, Horvitz HR. Genetic control of programmed cell death in the nematode C. elegans. Cell 1986;44:817–29.

26. Bakrania P, Efthymiou M, Klein JC, et al. Mutations in BMP4 cause eye, brain and digit developmental anomalies: overlap between BMP4 and hedgehog signaling pathways. Am J Hum Genet 2008;82: 304–19.

27. Malik S, Grzeschik KH. Synpolydactyly: clinical and molecular advances. Clin Genet 2008;73:113–20.

28. Paznekas WA, Boyadjiev SA, Shapiro RE, et al. Connexion 43 (GJA1) mutations cause the pleiotropic phenotype of oculodentodigitaldysplasia. Am J Hum Genet 2003;72:408–18.

29. Balk K, Biesecker LG. The clinical atlas of Greig cephalopolysyndactyly syndrome. Am J Med Genet A 2008;146A:548–57.

30. Mantilla-Capacho JM, Arnaud L, Diaz-Rodriguez, et al. Apert syndrome with preaxial polysyndactyly showing the typical mutation Ser252Trp in the FGFR2 gene. Genet Couns 2005;16:403–6.

31. Ibrahimi OA, Chiu ES, McCarthy JG, et al. Understanding the molecular basis of Apert syndrome. Plast Reconstr Surg 2005;115:264–70.

32. Witt PD, MacArthur CA. Molecular biology and congenital hand anomalies: from molecules and mutations to man. Plast Reconstr Surg 1998;102: 2254–67.

33. Buck-Gramcko D. Congenital malformations: syndactyly and related deformities. In: Nigst H, Buck-Gramcko D, Millesi H, et al, editors. Hand surgery. New York: Thieme Medical Publishers; 1988. p. 12.12.

34. Johannson S. Nagelwallbildung durch thernalappen bei kompletter syndacktylie. Handchirurgie 1982;14:199–203.

35. Johannson S. Nail folds in total syndactyly. Paper read at the First Congress of the International Federation of Societies for Surgery of the Hand, Rotterdam, June 16–20, 1980.

36. Hentz V. Correspondence newsletter. Rosemont (IL): American Society for Surgery of the Hand; 1985:65.

37. Sommerkamp T, Ezaki M, Carter PR, et al. A composite graft for complete syndactyly fingertip operations. J Hand Surg [Am] 1992;17:15–20.

38. Niranjan NS, De Carpentier J. A new technique for the division of syndactyly. Eur J Plast Surg 1990;13: 101–4.

39. Ekerot L. Syndactyly correction without skin-grafting. J Hand Surg [Br] 1996;21B:330–7.

40. Vickers D, Donnelly W. Corrective surgery of syndactyly without the use of skin grafts. Hand Surg 1996;1:203–9.

41. Eaton C, Lister GD. Syndactyly. Hand Clin 1990;6: 555–75.

42. Roswell A, Godfrey A. A fortuitous donor site for full thickness skin grafts in the correction of syndactyly. Br J Plast Surg 1984;37:31–4.

43. Park S, Hata Y, Ito E, et al. Full-thickness skin graft from the ulnar aspect of the wrist to cover defects on the hands and digits. Ann Plast Surg 1999;42: 129–31.

44. Zoltie N, Verlende P, Logan A. Full thickness grafts taken from the plantar instep for syndactyly release. J Hand Surg [Br] 1989;14:201–3.

45. Upton J. Congenital anomalies of the hand and forearm. In: May JW Jr, Littler JW, editors. The hand. In: McCarthy JG, editor. Plastic surgery, Vol 8. Philadelphia: WB Saunders; 1990. p. 5213–398.

46. Oates S, Gosain AK. Syndactyly repair performed simultaneously with circumcision: use of foreskin as a skin-graft donor site. J Pediatr Surg 1997;32:1482–4.

47. Benatar N. Full-thickness skin grafts from the cubital fossa for syndactyly release. Handchir Mikrochir Plast Chir 2004;35:186–8.

48. Sherif M. V-Y dorsal metacarpal flap: a new technique for the correction of syndactyly without skin graft. Plast Reconstr Surg 1998;101:1861–6.

49. Aydin A, Çelet Özden B. Dorsal metacarpal island flap in syndactyly treatment. Ann Plast Surg 2004;52:43–8.

50. Wafa AM. Hourglass dorsal metacarpal island flap: a new design for syndactylized web reconstruction. J Hand Surg 2008;33A:905–8.

51. Giele H, Rostek M. Syndactyly division without skin grafts by using dorsal flaps. In: Ogino T, editor. Congenital differences of the upper limb. Kyoto: Yamagata University School of Medicine; 2000. p. 78–80.

52. Ashmead D, Smith PJ. Tissue expansion for Apert's syndactyly. J Hand Surg [Br] 1995;20:327–30.

53. Ezaki M, Kay SPJ, Light TR, et al. Congenital hand deformities. In: Green D, Hotchkiss RN, Pederson WC, editors. Green's operative hand surgery, 4th edition, Vol 1. New York: Churchill Livingstone; 1999. p. 324–551.

54. Furnas D, Fischer G. The Z-plasty: biomechanics and mathematics. Br J Plast Surg 1971;24:144–60.

55. Woolf R, Broadbent T. The four-flap Z-plasty. Plast Reconstr Surg 1972;49:48–51.

56. Fereshetian S, Upton J. The anatomy and management of the thumb in Apert's syndrome. J Hand Surg [Am] 1982;7:450–3.

57. Foucher G, Medina J, Pajardi G, et al. Classification and treatment of symbrachydactyly. Chir Main 2000;19:161–8.

58. Buck-Gramcko D. Skin loss in the palm and web spaces. In: Evans D, editor. The hand and upper limb, Vol 9. Edinburgh: Churchill Livingstone; 1992. p. 159–80.

59. Buck-Gramcko D. Syndactyly between the thumb and index finger. In: Buck-Gramcko D, editor. Congenital malformations of the hand and forearm. London: Churchill Livingstone; 1998. p. 141–8.

60. Emmett A, Morris A. Ring constriction syndrome. In: Buck-Gramcko D, editor. Congenital malformations of the hand and forearm. London: Churchill Livingstone; 1998. p. 169–82.

61. Strauch B. Dorsal thumb flap for release of adduction contracture of the first web space. Bull Hosp Joint Dis 1975;36:34–9.

62. Flatt A, Wood VE. Multiple dorsal rotation flaps from the hand for thumb web contractures. Plast Reconstr Surg 1970;45:258–62.

63. Buck-Gramcko D. Angeborene fehlbildungen der hand. In: Nigst H, Buck-Gramcko D, Millesi H, et al, editors. Handchirurgie. New York: Thieme; 1988. p. 12.1–12.12 [in German].

64. Brown P. Adduction-flexion contracture of the thumb: correction with dorsal rotation flap and release of contracture. Clin Orthop 1972;88:161–8.

65. Caroli A, Zanasi S. First web space reconstruction by Caroli's technique in congenital hand deformities with severe thumb ray adduction. Br J Plast Surg 1989;42:653–9.

66. Sandzen S. Dorsal pedicle flap for resurfacing a moderate thumb index web contracture release. J Hand Surg Am 1982;7:24–7.

67. Zancolli E, Zancolli EJ. Congenital ulnar drift of the fingers. Hand Clin 1985;1:443–56.

68. Upton J, Coombes CJ, Havlik RJ. Use of forearm flaps for the severely contracted first web space in children with congenital malformations. J Hand Surg Am 1996;21:470–7.

69. Song R, Gao Y, Song Y, et al. The forearm flap. Clin Plast Surg 1982;9:21–6.

70. Masquelet AC, Penteado CV. Le lambeau interosseux posterieur. Ann Chir Main 1987;6:131–9.

71. Upton J. Classification and pathologic anatomy of limb anomalies. Clin Plast Surg 1991;18:321–56.

72. Kay S. Free tissue transfer in children. In: Gupta A, Kay SPJ, Scheker LR, editors. The growing hand: diagnosis and management of the upper extremity in children. London: CV Mosby; 2000. p. 969–86.

73. Muzaffar AR, Rafols F, Masson J, et al. Keloid formation after syndactyly reconstruction: associated conditions, prevalence and preliminary report of a treatment method. J Hand Surg Am 2004;29:201–8.

74. Tonkin MA, Willis KR, Lawson RD. Keloid formation resulting in acquired syndactyly of an initially normal web space following syndactyly release of an adjacent web space. J Hand Surg Eur Vol 2008;33:29–31.

75. Habenicht R. Web construction in complex syndactylies using soft tissue distraction. In: Ogino T, editor. Congenital differences of the upper limb. Kyoto: Yamagata University School of Medicine; 2000. p. 87–9.

76. Rider MA, Grindel SI, Tonkin MA, et al. An experience of the Snow-Littler procedure. J Hand Surg [Br] 2000;25:376–81.

77. Upton J. Management of transverse and longitudinal deficiencies (failure of formation). In:

Hentz VR, editor. The hand and upper limb (Part 2). In: Mathes SJ, editor. Plastic surgery, Vol 8. Philadelphia: Saunders Elsevier; 2006. p. 51–183.

78. Upton J. Constriction ring syndrome. In: Hentz VR, editor. The hand and upper limb (Part 2). In: Mathes SJ, editor. Plastic surgery, Vol 8. Philadelphia: Saunders Elsevier; 2006. p. 185–213.

79. Posch J, Dela Cruz-Saddal FA, Posch JL Jr. Congenital syndactylism of fingers in 262 cases. Orthop Rev 1981;10:23–32.

80. Losch G, Duncker H. Anatomy and surgical treatment of syndactyly. Plast Reconstr Surg 1972;50: 167–73.

81. Rolle A, Wilhelm K. Syndactylia results. Handchir Mikrochir Plast Chir 1984;16:52–5.

82. De Smet L, Van Ransbeeck H, Deneef G. Syndactyly release: results of the Flatt technique. Acta Orthop Belg 1998;64:301–5.

83. Keret D, Ger E. Evaluation of a uniform operative technique to treat syndactyly. J Hand Surg Am 1987;12:727–9.

84. Percival N, Sykes PJ. Syndactyly: a review of the factors which influence surgical treatment. J Hand Surg [Br] 1989;14:196–200.

85. Toledo L, Ger E. Evaluation of the operative treatment of syndactyly. J Hand Surg Am 1979;4: 556–64.

86. Dobyns J. Problems and complications in the management of upper limb anomalies. Hand Clin 1986;2:373–81.

87. Deutinger M, Mandl H, Frey M, et al. Late results following surgical correction of syndactyly and symbrachydactyly. Z Kinderchir 1989;44:50–4.

88. Meissl G, Millesi H, Piza-Katzer H. Critical considerations of various surgical methods for correction of syndactylia (report on an observation period of 10–20 years). Handchirurgie 1975;7: 69–75.

89. van der Biezen J, Bloem JJ. Dividing the fingers in congenital syndactyly release: a review of more than 200 years of surgical treatment. Ann Plast Surg 1994;33:225–30.

90. Blauth W. Syndaktylie und rezidiv. Fingersyndaktylien und ihre behandlung. Z Orthop Ihre Grenzgeb 1979;117:523–30.

91. Moss A, Foucher G. Syndactyly: can web creep be avoided? J Hand Surg [Br] 1990;15:193–200.

92. Marumo E, Kojima T, Suzuki S. An operation for syndactyly, and its results. Plast Reconstr Surg 1976;58:561–7.

93. Neff G, Plaue R, Aulbach D. Results of various operations for syndactylia follow-up studies and statistical evaluation of 101 primary operations. Handchirurgie 1978;10:21–30.

94. Brauer R, Cronin T, Smoot W. Treatment of syndactylism. In: Goldwyn R, editor. Long-term results in plastic and reconstructive surgery. Boston: Little, Brown; 1980. p. 812–35.

95. Eslov B, Zachariae L. Surgical methods in syndactylism. Acta Chir Scand 1966;131:258–326.

96. Bastian H, Schutze C. Results of surgical treatment of syndactylia of the hand. Beitr Orthop Traumatol 1989;36:267–74.

97. Bensahel H, Boureau M. Medecine pratique et syndactylies. Rev Prat 1972;22:3265–74.

98. Helbig B, Hippe P. Preliminary report of the results of syndactyly surgery. Handchir Mikrochir Plast Chir 1984;16:44–7.

99. Johne B. Operative behandlung der syndaktylie: zeitpunkt – technik – egrebnisse [thesis]. Hamburg University, Hamburg; 1979.

100. Kramer R, Hildreth DH, Brinker MR, et al. A comparison of patients with different types of syndactyly. J Pediatr Orthop 1998;18:233–8.

101. Ruby L, Goldberg M. Syndactyly and polydactyly. Orthop Clin North Am 1976;7:361–74.

102. Schrader M, Losch G. Differential diagnosis, operative treatment, and prognosis of complicated syndactylies. Handchir Mikrochir Plast Chir 1985; 17:122–8.

Failure of Differentiation: Part II (Arthrogryposis, Camptodactyly, Clinodactyly, Madelung Deformity, Trigger Finger, and Trigger Thumb)

Jennifer M. Ty, MD[a], Michelle A. James, MD[b,c],*

KEYWORDS

- Arthrogryposis • Camptodactyly • Clinodactyly
- Madelung deformity • Trigger finger • Trigger thumb

ARTHROGRYPOSIS

The term "arthrogryposis" has traditionally been used to describe various conditions that present with congenital joint contractures.[1] Under this broad term, more than 150 separate disease entities that share elements of congenital contractures have been described.[2] The contractures are considered to be the end result of decreased intra-uterine movement by the fetus after a period of normal development. This decreased movement may occur because of neuropathies, myopathies, abnormal connective tissue, or decreased intra-uterine space.[2]

Classic arthrogryposis or arthrogryposis multiplex congenita describes a specific disease process. This term was first used by Stern[3] to describe three children in 1923. To add to the terminological confusion, Sheldon[4] gave a detailed clinical description of this same entity in 1932 and called it amyoplasia or amyoplasia congenita, emphasizing his belief that the disease was the result of aplasia or hypoplasia of certain muscle groups. This article focuses on the cause and upper extremity treatment considerations of this disorder, which is referred to as amyoplasia.

Distal arthrogryposis refers to a large subgroup of disorders in which the contractures primarily involve the hands and feet. Multiple classification schemes have been used to describe these conditions, but this group is extremely heterogenous and this term does not refer to a specific disease entity.[5–7]

Children who have amyoplasia present with a characteristic phenotype at birth. Most (84%) present with involvement of all four limbs, although

[a] Hand and Upper Extremity Division, Department of Orthopaedic Surgery, Alfred I. duPont Hospital for Children, Nemours, 1600 Rockland Road, Room 1H-65C, Wilmington, DE 19803, USA
[b] Department of Orthopaedic Surgery, Shriners Hospital for Children Northern California, 2425 Stockton Boulevard, Sacramento CA 95817, USA
[c] Department of Orthopaedic Surgery, Division of Pediatric Orthopaedics, University of California Davis School of Medicine, 4860 Y Street, Suite 3800, Sacramento, CA 95817 USA
* Corresponding author. Department of Orthopaedic Surgery, Division of Pediatric Orthopaedics, University of California Davis School of Medicine, 4860 Y St. Suite 3800, Sacramento, CA 95817 USA
E-mail address: mjames@shrinenet.org (M. James).

Hand Clin 25 (2009) 195–213
doi:10.1016/j.hcl.2008.12.003

11% present with only lower limb involvement and 5% with only upper limb involvement.[8] The limbs appear fusiform and cylindric with a pronounced decrease in muscle mass and a lack of flexion creases. There is decreased joint range of motion with a firm inelastic endpoint.[9] Sensation is normal and there are few associated visceral anomalies. The joint contractures are usually bilaterally symmetric. The shoulders are internally rotated and adducted, the elbows are extended, the wrists are flexed and ulnarly deviated, the thumb is adducted, and the fingers are partially flexed.[9] The hips are often flexed and abducted, and one or both hips are dislocated in one third of patients.[10] Knee flexion contractures are the most common presentation, but the child may present with knee extension contractures, and knee joint subluxation or dislocation may be present. Almost all children who have this condition have rigid clubfeet, although congenital vertical talus or another foot deformity may be present. Congenital scoliosis is unusual and should trigger the work-up of other neuromuscular disorders. Neuromuscular scoliosis may develop in 30% of patients, however.[10] Some 90% of patients who have all four limbs involved have a characteristic frontal midline capillary hemangioma.[11]

Amyoplasia is sporadic, with an incidence of 1 of every 10,000 live births.[12] Fifteen identical twin cohorts have been reported in the literature as being discordant for the disease.[13] This finding strongly suggests that genetics do not play a major role in the disease, and that some factors in twins may contribute to the condition.[13] Several authors have primarily attributed amyoplasia to be the end result of damage to the anterior horn cells of the spinal cord.[14,15] Others believe that a primary myogenic form may exist.[12] Multiple studies have not found a clear environmental cause.[16]

Several authors have commented that children who have amyoplasia are often of above-average intelligence and have the potential to become independent adults despite significant physical limitations.[9,17] Bevan and colleagues[18] suggest that to help a child who has amyoplasia reach this goal, treatment should be focused on communication, activities of daily living, mobilization, and ambulation, in decreasing order of importance. With this in mind, treatment of the upper extremity must focus on preserving or increasing motion and allowing the upper extremities to be positioned at the tabletop level for self-care and access to computers.[17] Because children who have amyoplasia are extremely limited with regard to upper extremity strength, they depend on bimanual patterns and this must be preserved.[17] Van Heest and colleagues[19] reported one patient who had

a loss in function after the development of an elbow flexion contracture. This condition, combined with the patient's pre-existing contralateral elbow extension contracture, led to a decline in the ability to perform activities of daily living. Occupational therapy is often helpful in assisting with learning adaptive skills and providing assistive equipment.

Most frequently, the child who has upper extremity involvement benefits from treatment of elbow and wrist contractures. The typical arthrogrypotic deformity of the elbows is full extension with some triceps function.[17] The lack of passive elbow flexion is particularly disabling because it does not allow hand-to-mouth function. Children who have amyoplasia who have passive elbow flexion but lack active flexion are often able to use strategies, such as trunk swaying or table top propping, to flex the elbow for self-feeding.[20] Tendon transfers to restore active flexion of the elbow are difficult given the relative lack of donor musculature and carry a significant risk for creating an elbow flexion contracture. They seem to provide little additional functional benefit for most children who have amyoplasia.[20]

Initial treatment of the upper extremities in the infant who has amyoplasia begins with gentle manipulation and splinting. This treatment may be particularly helpful with regard to the wrist flexion and elbow extension contractures. Therapy may also assist in maintaining muscle mass and strength in the child who has amyoplasia.[21] Smith and Drennan[22] evaluated 17 infants who had wrist flexion contractures and found that patients who had distal arthrogryposis were more responsive to early casting, serial casting, and orthotics than patients who had amyoplasia.

Timing of upper extremity surgery is controversial. Mennen advocated an early one-stage corrective procedure between 3 and 6 months of age.[23] He recommended proximal row carpectomy to address the wrist flexion contracture and the triceps-to-radius transfer to achieve active elbow flexion. In his report on 47 limbs, he found that patients who were operated on early gained more active motion and had improved carpal bone remodeling. He also believed that the repositioning the wrist allowed for improved finger function and noted that creases developed over the finger joints after wrist surgery.

Because amyoplasia frequently involves all four extremities, however, some advocate waiting until the child begins to ambulate before beginning upper extremity surgery. This recommendation may result in a significant time delay, given that clubfeet, knee contractures, and hip dislocations often need to be addressed. In the nonambulatory or ambulate-with-assist child, there were concerns regarding maintaining elbow extension to allow transfers and crutch or walker use. Van Heest and colleagues[19] reported a series of patients treated with triceps-to-biceps transfers and did not find that the associated loss of active extension strength or the development of elbow flexion contractures affected mobility.

Van Heest recommended elbow capsulotomy with triceps lengthening at 18 to 24 months of age if the child does not achieve 90° of passive elbow flexion following a minimum of 6-month stretching program.[19] Ezaki[17] reports a preference for beginnning upper extremity operative procedures before age 4 because children often have developed well-adapted use patterns by age 8 that may be disrupted by surgical changes in the upper extremity positioning. In addition, operations may be coordinated with lower extremity procedures to decrease the total number of operations.

Van Heest and colleagues[20] reported their experience with posterior elbow capsulotomy with triceps lengthening in their series of 29 elbows in 23 children with a mean follow up of 5.4 years. The arc of motion improved from an average of 32° to 66°. All children were able to get their hands to their mouths using passive assistance techniques, such as cross-arm, table-push, and trunk-sway. A total of 22 of the 23 children were able to feed independently; the remaining child was limited by poor hand function. Preoperatively, only 2 children were able to demonstrate measurable biceps function. At final follow-up, 7 children had some biceps function, suggesting that allowing passive elbow motion may have unmasked biceps function in some patients.

Restoring active elbow flexion in children who have amyoplasia is difficult, and as Van Heest and colleagues[20] have shown, possibly not necessary. Unless the child has good passive elbow flexion and a strong muscle available for transfer, which are unusual conditions in these patients, the results of elbow flexion transfers are disappointing and if unopposed, tend to cause severe flexion contractures.

Van Heest and colleagues[19] also reported their experience with tendon transfers with and without posterior elbow releases to restore active elbow flexion. Although they believed triceps-to-biceps tendon transfer gave the most predictable results, patients developed flexion contractures, with an average flexion contracture of 38°. Five patients underwent a bipolar pectoralis major and four underwent a latissimus dorsi transfer. Although both operations have the theoretic advantage of adding muscle to the arm, both donor muscles are difficult to test preoperatively, require extensive surgical dissection, and yield disappointing results. Van Heest now recommends against active elbow flexion transfers in this population, because children are able to passively flex the elbow against their leg or a table top to perform activities of daily living.[20]

Steindler flexorplasty has been considered contraindicated by many authors because of a theoretical risk for worsening the typical wrist palmar flexion and pronation deformity by moving the flexor pronator origin proximally. Goldfarb and colleagues[24] reported promising results in 17 elbows in 10 children treated with Steindler flexorplasty, however. The flexor pronator origin was isolated and transferred to the anterior humerus approximately 2 to 3 cm proximal to the medial epicondyle with the elbow flexed at 80°. Postoperatively, all elbows had active flexion against gravity to 85°. They did note that patients developed a mean elbow flexion contracture of 28° and that the total arc of pronation and supination decreased from a mean of 88° to 41°. They did not find an increase in wrist flexion or finger flexion posture after surgery, however.

The arthrogrypotic flexed and ulnar deviated wrist often benefits from repositioning in a more functional neutral position. Proximal row carpectomy,[23,25] dorsal radial wedge resection osteotomy,[26] and arthrodesis[27] at maturity have all been advocated. All of these present difficulties, however. Proximal row carpectomy may not provide adequate wrist extension and wrist motion may not be maintained. Dorsal radial wedge resection is frequently not at the point of maximum deformity and may jeopardize growth at the distal radius along with radiocarpal motion. Arthrodesis at maturity eliminates all wrist motion.

Ezaki and Carter[17,28] have described a technique of dorsal carpal wedge osteotomy that reduces the deformity while retaining motion at the radiocarpal joint (Fig. 1). A volar approach is first performed to release the tight forearm fascia and the wrist flexor tendons are released or lengthened. From a separate dorsal incision, the wrist extensors are isolated, and a biplanar dorsal radial wedge of carpus is resected taking care to protect the radiocarpal articulation. The osteotomy is closed and the extensor carpi ulnaris is transferred to the extensor carpi radialis. In 42 wrists in 24 patients with an average follow-up of 18 months,[28] the resting position of the wrist improved from 59° of flexion to 11° with a more centered arc of motion.

Although the shoulder has limited motion and often has an internal rotation contracture, this is usually not functionally limiting. Patients who

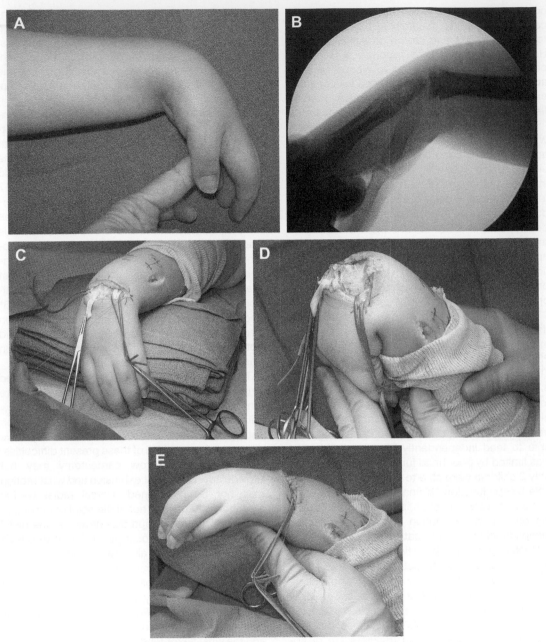

Fig. 1. Dorsal carpal wedge osteotomy for wrist flexion contracture in child who has amyoplasia. (*A*) Preoperative clinical photograph. (*B*) Intraoperative radiograph with wrist in maximum passive extension. (*C*) Transverse incision over dorsal carpal row. Extensor carpi radialis brevis (in clamp) sectioned proximally. Extensor carpi ulnaris (in vessel loop) prepared for later transfer. (*D*) Proximal cut made at the level of the capsular attachment of the proximal carpal row perpendicular to long axis of the forearm. Distal cut through the distal carpal row perpendicular to the long axis of the metacarpals. (*E*) Alignment after closing wedge osteotomy.

have extreme internal rotation may benefit from an external rotation humeral osteotomy to place them in a resting position of 45° of internal rotation to allow midline function.[17] The thumb-in-palm deformity may require a thenar release in which the origins of the abductor pollicis brevis, the opponens pollicis, flexor pollicis brevis, and both heads of the adductor pollicis are released.[17] Skin deficiency is usually palmar, at the level of the thumb metacarpophalangeal joint; this benefits more from a rotation flap from the radial side of the index finger than from a first web z-plasty.[17]

Finger motion usually does not benefit from direct surgical treatment, although some have reported improved function after wrist repositioning.[23]

CAMPTODACTYLY

Camptodactyly is a nontraumatic, often progressive flexion contracture of the proximal interphalangeal joint (PIPJ) that usually affects the little finger. Since Tamplin's original description in 1846,[29] there has been much debate regarding the definition, etiology, and treatment of camptodactyly. The true incidence of camptodactyly is unclear, especially when mild cases may go unreported, but it is estimated to affect less than 1% of the population.[30]

Benson and colleagues[31] combined elements of earlier classification systems and described camptodactyly as falling into three main categories. Type I, or classic camptodactyly, presents in infancy. Frequently, the disorder is confined to one or both little fingers. The ring and long fingers may also be involved, however. Males and females seem to be affected equally.[32] This type of camptodactyly is usually sporadic, but it may be inherited as an autosomal dominant trait with incomplete penetrance.[29]

Type II shares similar clinical characteristics to type I, but presents in adolescence. Females seem to be more often affected than males (**Fig. 2**). The deformity tends to worsen with the adolescent growth spurt.[29] Because infancy and adolescence are normal times of rapid growth, this may account for the bimodal distribution.

Type III is a more severe form of camptodactyly (**Fig. 3**). In this variant, severe flexion contractions are seen usually involving multiple digits of both hands.[33] This form of camptodactyly is associated with other congenital anomalies. Multiple

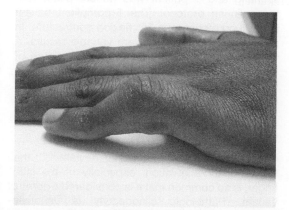

Fig. 2. Type II camptodactyly. This patient also had postaxial polydactyly treated in infancy.

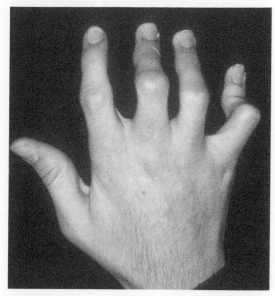

Fig. 3. Type III camptodactyly with multiple finger involvement.

chromosomal disorders, craniofacial diseases, and skeletal deformities have been associated with camptodactyly. The occurrence of type III camptodactyly follows the inheritance pattern of the specific disorder with which it is associated.

There is no consensus regarding the causative etiology of camptodactyly, and essentially all structures about the PIPJ have been implicated in the disorder.[34] Many anatomic differences have been noted in digits with camptodactyly, and it is difficult to determine which are causative factors and which are secondary changes as a result of the development of the contracture.

Multiple authors have attributed the deformity to a generalized imbalance between the flexor and the extensor tendons leading to secondary contractures.[34,35] McFarlane[36] argues that camptodactyly is an intrinsic minus deformity condition caused specifically by an abnormal lumbrical insertion (most frequently into the MPJ capsule). Others have noted frequent abnormalities with regard to the flexor digitorum superficialis (FDS) length or an anomalous origin of the FDS from the palmar fascia or transverse ligament.[29,37] Still others have argued that the causes are tightness of the skin and connective tissues,[38] malposition of the extensor lateral bands,[39] or contractures of the joint itself.[40] With the development of a flexion contracture, abnormal tension on the extensor mechanism may further contribute to the deformity.[41] In addition to soft tissue anomalies, camptodactyly may be associated with changes in bony anatomy with flattening of the proximal phalanx head and the base of the middle phalanx, and an indentation along the proximal phalanx neck. These are generally regarded to be secondary changes, however. Smith and Grobbelaar[41] took a more global approach and argued that all of the described anatomic factors occur to various degrees in all patients and that in particular, the fascial structures, lumbricals, and FDS tendon are nearly always involved.

The effectiveness of treatment of camptodactyly is difficult to assess from the literature. Some series include different types of camptodactyly, and criteria for success vary among studies. Authors who have identified a specific causative factor have tended to argue for surgical treatment to address the particular anatomic issue. Others who emphasize a generalized imbalance as causative have recommended splinting with good success. Many note that full flexion, especially of the ulnar digits, is more important than extension and have cautioned against aggressive treatment to address the lack of full extension at the risk of compromising the ability to fully flex the digits. All have noted that surgical treatment is associated with decreased motion of the PIPJ.

Some have argued for conservative management with splinting regimens in nearly all cases.[31,42] Other have promoted more aggressive operative management,[37,43] particularly citing difficulties with compliance with splinting regimens in the adolescent age group.

Smith and Kaplan recommended an FDS tenotomy.[29] They reported a decrease in the flexion deformity of at least 33% in 12 fingers that were treated in this manner. McFarlane and colleagues[43] believed that it was critical to address the anomalous insertion of the lumbrical and the resultant intrinsic minus hand position by releasing the lumbrical and performing an FDS tendon transfer to the extensor mechanism. In their series of 53 patients with 1 year follow-up, they found that the joint contracture was reduced from a mean of 49° to a mean of 25°. They did note that patients had a slow return of flexion, however, and that only 33% of patients regained full flexion at 1 year with an average residual lag of 1.8 cm from the distal palmar crease. Gupta and Burke[34] recommended extensor indicis proprius transfer to the radial extensor expansion to improve intrinsic function.

Smith and Grobbelaar[41] reported on their experience on 18 fingers in 16 patients. They released tight soft tissues and abnormal lumbrical insertions, lengthened the FDS, and splinted the patients in extension for 4 weeks to address the lax extensor mechanism. They reported 15 patients had good to excellent results. Three patients who had preoperative bony changes of the proximal phalanx did poorly. Siegert and colleagues[44] reported their results with both nonoperative (38 fingers in 21 patients) and operative (41 fingers in 14 patients) treatment. Their operation was individualized, but most patients underwent a release of the FDS. Additional soft tissue procedures were performed in a smaller percentage of patients. In their operative group, only 7 fingers were rated as good, and there were no excellent results. They noted an average improvement in the flexion contracture of only 10°, and 10 patients were noted to have lost considerable flexion. Of their nonoperatively treated patients, 12 patients had improvements in extension and only two had loss of flexion.

Hori and colleagues[42] reported on 34 fingers in 24 patients. They recommended wearing a dynamic Capener-type splint for 24 hours a day for several months, followed by maintenance splinting of 8 hours per day. They reported that 20 fingers showed almost full correction of the flexion contracture, 9 fingers were improved, 3 fingers were unchanged, and 2 fingers worsened. They did note recurrence if the splinting was discontinued and recommended continuing splinting indefinitely until full growth. Benson and colleagues[31] reported results on 59 fingers in 22 patients with a mean follow-up of 33 months. This group was divided into 13 patients who had type I deformities, 4 patients who had type II deformities, and 5 patients who had type III deformities. Patients were treated with a nighttime progressive extension splinting program. They found splinting to be particularly effective in type I camptodactyly in which patients improved from an average flexion contracture of 23° to 4°, and 18 of the 24 PIPJs achieved full passive extension. Two of the type II patients requested operative intervention because they were unwilling to participate in splinting and 1 patient was noncompliant with the splinting protocol. The 1 compliant patient had full correction of a 35° flexion contracture. In the type III group, there were variable results. A total of 12 fingers with a flexion contracture of greater than or equal to 15° improved to almost full extension, and 2 patients underwent surgical correction for severe contractures.

CLINODACTYLY

Clinodactyly refers to radioulnar deviation of the finger. Minor angulation, especially of the little finger, is so common that it is considered a normal variant. Pathologic clinodactyly is variously described as greater than 10°[45] or 15°[46] of angulation (Fig. 4A).

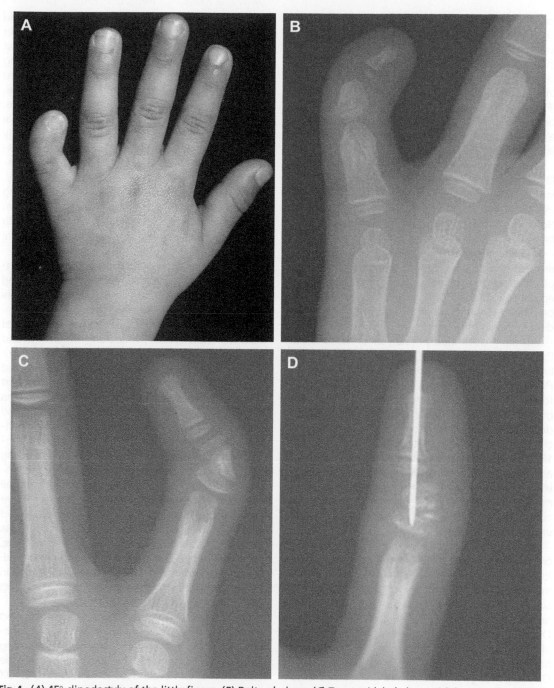

Fig. 4. (*A*) 45° clinodactyly of the little finger. (*B*) Delta phalanx. (*C*) Trapezoidal phalanx with longitudinal epiphyseal bracket. (*D*) Closing wedge osteotomy in the same patient.

Clinodactyly of the little finger is inherited in an autosomal dominant fashion and usually presents bilaterally.[47] Estimates regarding the incidence of clinodactyly range from 1% to 20%.[48] The next most common sites of occurrence are the thumb and ring finger, with involvement of the middle and index fingers being relatively uncommon.[49]

Clinodactyly may also be associated with other hand anomalies and syndromic conditions.[50]

The deformity is usually caused by an abnormally shaped middle phalanx, which may be triangular or trapezoidal because of a C-shaped physis extending from the normal proximal physis along the shortened side of the phalanx and connecting to an often aberrantly persistent distal physis.[51] Light and Ogden[52] have further characterized the longitudinal epiphyseal bracket responsible for this and other angular deformities. Early complete ossification of the bracket leads to a very short triangular "delta" phalanx and angular deformity (**Fig. 4**B), whereas an incomplete or cartilaginous bracket allows some longitudinal growth causing a trapezoidal phalanx and the resultant digit angulation (**Fig. 4**C).

Most cases of clinodactyly, especially of the little finger, do not require treatment because there is little functional impairment and surgical treatment carries a risk for scarring and stiffness. Splinting and therapy have not been advocated because of lack of efficacy.[52]

Surgical correction has been recommended for severe clinodactyly. Operative treatment consists of either segmental resection of the longitudinal epiphyseal bracket to allow for correction with continued longitudinal growth or an osteotomy to directly realign the digit.

Vickers[53] described physiolysis or resection of the mid-zone of the longitudinal epiphyseal bracket with a fat interposition graft in 6 patients. Postoperative splinting was not required, and he found improvement in length and angulation with growth. Caouette-Laberge and colleagues[54] described their experience with 35 fingers in 23 children and found a mean angular correction of 18° in children who had surgery before 6 years of age. Fingers with more severe preoperative angulation (greater than 40°) were observed to have more significant angular correction (mean 20°) compared with fingers with less than 40° of preoperative angulation (mean 7.5°).

Closing wedge, opening wedge, and combined or "reverse" osteotomies have all been advocated for surgical correction. Closing wedge osteotomies have the advantage of relative technical simplicity, but carry the risk for further shortening an already shortened digit (**Fig. 4**D).[50] Light and Ogden pointed out that a reverse osteotomy may allow the formation of a bony bridge that crosses both physes and thus limits further growth.[52] Opening wedge and combined procedures allow for length maintenance, but may require extensive dissection or local soft tissue rearrangement.[55,56]

MADELUNG DEFORMITY

In 1878, Madelung described the wrist deformity that bears his name at the Congress of German Society for Surgery in Berlin.[57] It had previously been noted by other surgeons, including Dupuytren, in the mid-1800s. The clinical manifestation is of a shortened radius and increased palmar and ulnar tilt of the radial articular surface. The relatively normal ulna is prominent dorsally, and the carpus is volar and ulnarly subluxed.[58] Wrist extension and supination are limited. Madelung deformity seems to be the result of the premature closure of the palmar and ulnar distal radial physis. Rarely, a reverse Madelung pattern presents, associated with dorsal-ulnar distal radial physeal arrest with dorsal hand displacement and a volarly prominent ulna. There is currently much discussion regarding the genetics, radiographic assessment, and treatment of Madelung deformity. There is some debate as to whether Madelung deformity represents an isolated disease process. Madelung deformity has been associated with repetitive loading of the wrist leading to a partial physeal arrest.[59]

The relationship of Madelung deformity to Leri-Weill dyschondrosteosis is also debated. Leri and Weill first described the dyschondrosteosis that bears their name in an article in 1929.[60] Leri-Weill dyschondrosteosis is a syndrome that includes short stature, Madelung deformity, and mesomelia or shortening of the middle segment of the extremities. Several authors have argued that Madelung deformity always presents as part of Leri-Weill dyschondrosteosis.[60] Other studies have concluded that patients who have isolated Madelung deformity may represent a discrete heritable condition.[58,61] Zebala and colleagues[58] reported that 17 of 22 of their cases of Madelung deformity fit the description of Leri-Weill dyschondrosteosis and argued that most but not all patients who have Madelung deformity have Leri-Weill dyschondrosteosis. They provided evidence that Madelung deformity presents as a spectrum that may affect only the distal radius, or the entire radius may be bowed and shortened. Madelung deformity is four times more common in females and most patients who have Madelung deformity present with bilateral changes.[60]

Belin and colleagues[62,63] and Shears and colleagues independently identified loss of function mutations in the short homeobox containing gene (SHOX) resulting in haploinsufficiency to be causative of Leri-Weill dyschondrosteosis. SHOX is located on the pseudoautosomal region of the X or Y chromosome, and has also been implicated in causing the short stature seen in Turner syndrome.[64] Mutations in both SHOX genes seems to result in Langer mesomelic dysplasia.[62] Estrogen may play a role in the development of Madelung deformity because this disease frequently presents in females at the time of adolescence. Madelung deformity is relatively uncommon, occurring only in 7% of patients who have Turner syndrome, a condition in which there is also SHOX haploinsufficiency and short stature.[65] Although some have postulated that the relative decrease in sex hormones seen in Turner syndrome may be protective, the loss of other modifying growth genes on the X chromosome may also play a role.[64] Genetic testing can be performed on patients to evaluate the SHOX gene. The SHOX gene and its developmental manifestations are continuing topics of ongoing research with many clinical implications.

Munns and colleagues[66] have found disorganization of the chondrocytes and abnormal endochondral calcification in the involved physis. SHOX has also been found to be expressed in the hypertropic chondrocytes of the growth plate and is believed to modulate cellular proliferation and viability.[67]

Vickers[68] noted the presence of an abnormal ligament between the anterior ulnar metaphysis of the distal radius and the carpus. This condensation of soft tissues begins in the volar metaphyseal region of the radius and attaches to the lunate and triangular fibrocartilage complex. There is sometimes an associated bone spur and fossa at the origin. This ligamentous structure has been noted histologically to have areas of fibrous tissue and fibrocartilage.[69] Murphy and colleagues[70] noted abnormalities in the pronator quadratus insertion. Others believe that these structures may merely represent a soft tissue compensatory response because of the need to support the carpus as a result of the abnormal growth of the radius and progressive loss of lunate facet support (H.R. McCarroll, MD, Sacramento CA, personal communication, August 2008). It is currently unclear if Vickers ligament contributes to the Madelung deformity or whether it is simply a secondary response of the soft tissues.

Imaging of the Madelung deformity can be difficult given that it is a complex three-dimensional deformity. The distal radius articular surface is flexed and pronated. Two-dimensional radiographs merely approximate the disease and must by taken in a uniform fashion to be helpful. Carter and Ezaki[69] describe a standardized fashion of obtaining a true posteroanterior (PA) view with neutral forearm rotation in which the patient kneels with the shoulder abducted and the elbow flexed 90°. They recommend having bilateral images on the same plate for ease of comparison.

Dannenberg and colleagues[71] described 12 radiographic criteria for the diagnosis of Madelung deformity. Several other researchers have attempted to define measurements based on the distal radius[72,73] but did not present reliability or reproducibility data for these measurements. Given

the significant changes in the radius in severe Madelung deformity, the usual bony landmarks are difficult to identify and the bowing of the distal radius makes the longitudinal axis of the radius difficult to determine. This difficulty limits the reproducibility of radially based measurements.

McCarroll and colleagues[74] identified four reliable and reproducible measurements for quantifying the severity of Madelung deformity on radiographs (**Fig. 5**). Tuder and colleagues[75] further evaluated these criteria and found significant correlations between the measurements. McCarroll and colleagues[76] have recently presented data comparing these measurements in normal wrists and wrists with Madelung deformity. They found that an ulnar tilt of greater than 28°, lunate subsistence of greater than 3 mm, and palmar carpal displacement of greater than 19 mm only occurred in wrists with Madelung deformity. In addition, they found the lunate fossa angle measurement to have the least overlap with normal wrists, which may represent an early radiographic finding of Madelung deformity.

Treatment of Madelung deformity is controversial. As McCarroll notes, there has been little documentation in studies of treatment of Madelung deformity that the severity of pain, altered range of motion, or visual deformity correlates to the degree of bony deformity.[74] The natural history of the disorder is not clearly understood, and it is not clear if the deformity is always associated with pain or functional limitation. Some argue that the most common reason for surgery is appearance, because most patients dislike the radial bowing and dorsal ulnar prominence.[77] Many adolescents and adults who have Madelung deformity complain of ulnar wrist pain, which may represent a degree of ulnocarpal impingement.[78,79]

Because the natural history is not clearly understood, it is difficult to recommend a course of treatment in the younger, asymptomatic patient. There is also debate regarding whether intervention can prevent the development of deformity. Vickers reported a reduction in pain and an improvement in the appearance of the wrist with growth in his series of patients who underwent surgical physiolysis, and in fact titled his report "Surgical prophylaxis (physiolysis) during the late growth period by resection of the dyschondrosteosis lesion."[68] In contrast, Carter and Ezaki[69] reported that they had limited success with epiphysiolysis. They attributed this in part to their Madelung deformity patient population generally presenting in late adolescence, a point at which they had limited remaining growth potential of the distal radius.

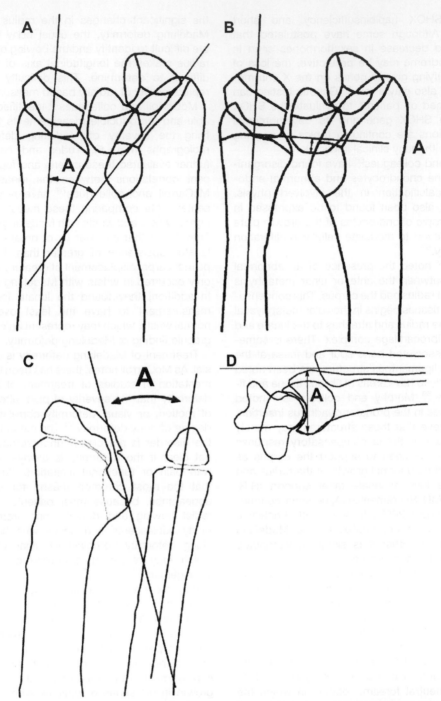

Fig. 5. (*A*) Ulnar tilt on a PA radiograph is defined as the complement of the acute angle (angle A) between the longitudinal axis of the ulna and a line tangent to the proximal surfaces of the scaphoid and lunate. (*B*) Lunate subsidence on a PA radiograph (distance A) is defined as the distance in millimeters between the most proximal point of the lunate and a line perpendicular to the longitudinal axis of the ulna and through its distal articular surface. The measurement is positive if the ulna exceeds distal to the proximal surface of the lunate. (*C*) Lunate fossa angle on a PA radiograph is defined as the complement of the acute angle (angle A) between the longitudinal axis of the ulna and a line across the lunate fossa of the radius. (*D*) Palmar carpal displacement on a lateral radiograph (distance A) is defined as the distance in millimeters between the longitudinal axis of the ulna and the most palmar point on the surface of the lunate or capitate. (*From* McCarroll HR, James MA, Newmeyer WL, et al. Madelung's deformity: quantitative assessment of x-ray deformity. J Hand Surg [Am] 2005;30(6):1213–4; with permission.)

Carter and Ezaki[69] have described their technique combining a release of Vickers ligament with a dome osteotomy by way of an anterior approach on 23 wrists in 18 patients (**Fig. 6**). They found that simple release of Vickers ligament may be helpful in alleviating pain; many patients reported improvement in their symptoms even before their osteotomy had healed. In addition, they found that release of this ligament allowed the carpus to assume a more normal alignment on the radius.[69,80] The same group later reported on their results on 26 wrists in 18 patients treated with a volar Vickers ligament release and dome osteotomy. Patients reported decreased pain and improved appearance, which was associated with radiographic changes in the mean radial inclination and lunate subsidence. There was persistent ulnocarpal and distal radial ulnar joint deformity, however.[81]

Many other procedures have been described for the treatment of Madelung deformity. Initially, treatment tended to focus on removal of the prominent ulna. Since Ranawat reported that the carpus tended to sublux ulnarly in wrists treated with an isolated Darrach procedure, however, this has fallen out of favor.[82] More recently the isolated ulnar wedge osteotomy or ulnar shortening osteotomy has been described for the treatment of mild Madelung deformity.[79,83]

Dos Reis and colleagues[73] described a dorsal closing wedge osteotomy of the distal radius combined with ulnar shortening, whereas Murphy and colleagues[70] and de Paula and colleagues[84] described a radial opening wedge osteotomy. Proponents have reported the successful correction of Madelung deformity using the Ilizarov technique.[85] Radial osteotomy and the Sauvé-Kapandji technique have also been described for the treatment of Madelung deformity.[86,87]

A recent English-language literature search found only two studies published on the long-term results after operatively treated Madelung deformity. Potenza and colleagues[88] published their results on 9 wrists in 5 patients with a mean follow-up of 34 years after surgery and a mean age at follow-up of 53 years. Eight wrists were treated operatively with a dorsoradially based closing wedge osteotomy, and either a shortening osteotomy of the distal ulna (six wrists) or a distal ulna resection (two wrists). All patients were noted to be pain-free and pleased with the cosmetic appearance of their operated wrists at follow-up. One patient who had a bilateral deformity who had elected to only have surgery on one wrist complained of pain in the unoperated wrist. Salon and colleagues[72] reported a mean 9.7 year follow-up on 11 wrists in 7 patients who were treated with

a similar dorsoradial closing wedge osteotomy and ulnar shortening osteotomy. All wrists were pain-free with daily activities and showed improved cosmetic appearance. Eight wrists showed remodeling of the distal radioulnar joint.

TRIGGER FINGER

Pediatric trigger fingers are uncommon and seem to represent a different entity from both pediatric trigger thumbs and adult trigger fingers. A unifying cause has not been determined in pediatric trigger finger. Instead, multiple anatomic anomalies, including an abnormal relationship between the FDS and the flexor digitorum profundus (FDP), an unusually proximal decussation of the FDS, nodules in the FDS or FDP, calcific tendonitis, mucopolysaccharidosis, and constriction of the A2 or A3 pulleys, have been identified in the literature.[89–92] Unlike trigger thumbs, which usually present with a fixed flexion deformity, trigger fingers are more likely to present with locking and catching symptoms.

In contrast to trigger digits in adults, isolated A1 pulley release is unlikely to successfully treat pediatric trigger fingers, because the triggering frequently does not occur at the A1 pulley (**Fig. 7**A). Tordai and Engkvist recommended additional procedures, such as widening of the FDS chiasm or partial division of the A2 pulley, for persistent triggering after A1 pulley release.[93] Cardon and colleagues[89] recommended an extensile approach to examine and also address other elements, including FDS slip resection.

Bae and colleagues[90] described their experience with 23 trigger fingers in 18 patients. All patients were treated with a standardized approach in which an A1 pulley release was performed by way of a Bruner-type incision and then a single slip of the FDS tendon was resected (**Fig. 7**B). This combination of procedures successfully resolved triggering in 91% of fingers. Two patients had recurrent triggering. One improved with a second procedure to resect the remaining FDS tendon slip, and the other was found to have an aberrant FDS muscle attachment that was released at the time of reoperation.

In our recent experience with a 17-month-old patient who had bilateral long finger trigger fingers, we found persistent bilateral intraoperative triggering despite a resection of the ulnar slip of the FDS tendon after an A1 pulley release. It was necessary to open the tendon sheath through a transverse incision just distal to the A2 pulley to complete the resection of the ulnar slip of the FDS tendon. After this was performed, there was

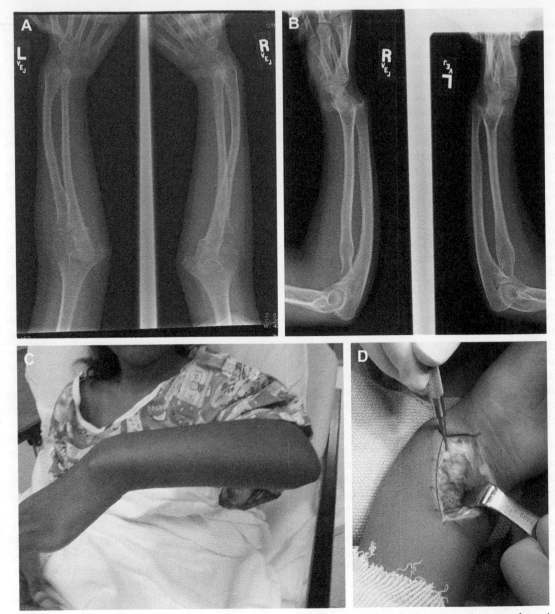

Fig. 6. Madelung deformity treated with a dome osteotomy and Vickers ligament resection by way of a volar approach. (*A*) Preoperative anteroposterior (AP) radiograph. (*B*) Preoperative lateral radiograph. (*C*) Preoperative clinical photograph. (*D*) Pronator quadratus and flexor carpi ulnaris retracted ulnarly. Probe is under Vickers ligament. (*E*) Vickers ligament resected (in forceps). Origin and fossa visible. (*F*) Dome osteotomy and translation of distal fragment using preplaced K-wire for control. (*G*) Postoperative AP radiograph. (*H*) Postoperative lateral radiograph. (*I*) Postoperative clinical photograph.

no longer any intraoperative evidence of triggering.

TRIGGER THUMB

Congenital trigger thumb is a controversial topic with varying opinions. Bae[94] recently performed an excellent evidence-based review of the literature and concluded that the natural history and recommended treatment remain unclear.

First, many consider the term "congenital" to be a misnomer. Although Dinham and Meggitt[95] reported 19 of 105 patients had a trigger thumb deformity at birth, this was on the basis of parental recall interviews. Several recent studies with physician examination of thousands of newborns

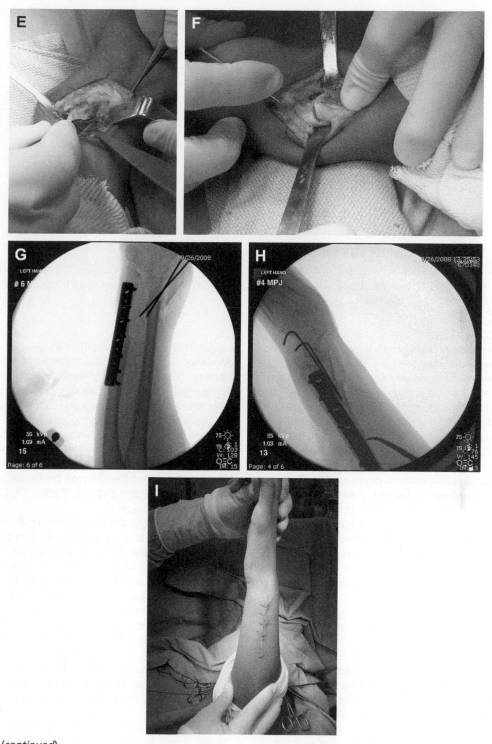

Fig. 6. (*continued*)

support the conclusion that trigger thumbs are an acquired condition. In the Rodgers and Waters study of 1046 newborns, the Slakey and Hennrikus study of 4719 newborns, and the Kikucki and

Ogino study of 1116 newborns, no cases of congenital trigger thumb were identified.[96–98]

Unlike adults who present with an intermittent locking or catching of the interphalangeal joint,

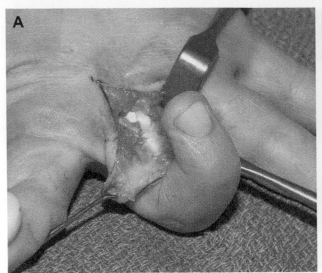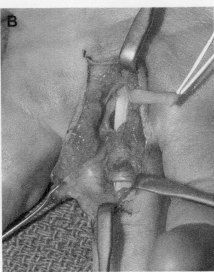

Fig. 7. Long trigger finger. (*A*) A1 pulley has been released, able to demonstrate continued triggering. (*B*) Ulnar slip of FDS resected (in forceps).

children usually present with the characteristic Notta nodule (thickening of the flexor pollicis longus tendon at the base of the metacarpophalangeal joint [MPJ] as originally described in 1850)[99] and a fixed flexion deformity of the interphalangeal joint (IPJ) (**Fig. 8**).[100] A smaller percentage may present with inability to actively flex the IPJ, when the thickened nodule is trapped distal to the A1 pulley. In a recent review of the literature, Ogino presents the classification scheme developed by Sugimoto and colleagues (originally published in Japanese).[101,102] In stage I, Notta nodule is present, but there is no triggering. In stage II, triggering is observed when the IPJ is actively extended. In stage III, the IPJ cannot be extended actively and triggering is observed when the IPJ is extended passively. In stage IV, the IPJ cannot be passively extended.

Although authors have speculated that thumb sucking or the characteristic thumb-in-fist grasp positioning of the infant incites localized trauma that leads to triggering,[103] this is not fully supported by pathologic studies. Electron microscopy examination of tendon nodules and sheaths from children who had trigger thumbs has not found evidence of degenerative or inflammatory changes.[104]

Trigger thumb occurrence is usually sporadic. Reports of trigger thumbs occurring in twins,[105] the frequent bilateral nature of the condition,[95] and the association of trigger thumb with congenital conditions, notably trisomy 13,[100] support a possible hereditary component, however. Shim and colleagues[106] reported a pedigree in which trigger thumbs were inherited in an autosomal dominant mode with incomplete penetrance. Because of the usual infant thumb-in-fist posturing, the precise development of this disorder can be difficult to determine. Kikuchi and Ogino[98] reported the prevalence of acquired trigger thumb at 1 year of age to be 3 per 1000 live births. In a retrospective review of 89 surgical trigger thumb releases performed in a 3-year period, Rodgers and Waters[96] found that none of the children presented at less than 3 months of age and only 6 presented at less than 6 months of age.

Like the etiology, the natural history of pediatric trigger thumbs is also unclear. In Dinham and Meggitt's[95] review, 30% of patients presenting soon after birth had a spontaneous recovery and no patient who was less than 3 years of age at the time of surgical release had a loss of IPJ motion. More recently, Baek and colleagues[107] reported in their prospective observational study of 71 trigger thumbs in 53 patients that 63% resolved spontaneously at an average age of 5 years; resolution was defined as a lack of IPJ flexion contracture. A subset of these patients had less IPJ hyperextension than their unaffected thumb, however.

Nonoperative management of pediatric trigger thumb may include extension exercises and splinting. Watanbe and colleagues[108] studied 58 thumbs in 46 children who were treated by daily passive extension exercises and found that 96% had satisfactory results. Final motion was abnormal in 59% of thumbs, however. Lee and colleagues[109] demonstrated improvement in

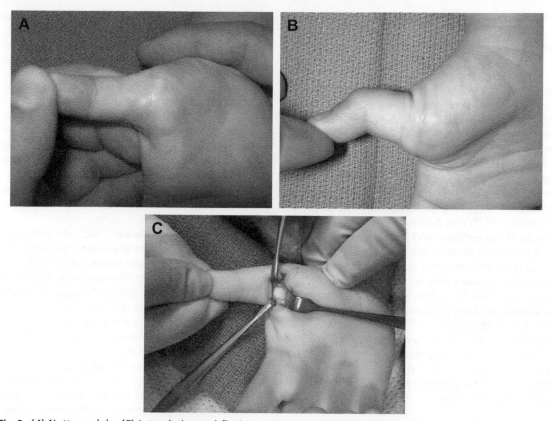

Fig. 8. (*A*) Notta nodule. (*B*) Interphalangeal flexion contracture. (*C*) Notta nodule intraoperative photograph.

flexion contractures in 71% of 31 thumbs using a protocol of full-time hyperextension splinting for 6 to 12 weeks followed by nighttime splinting.

Surgical release of the A1 pulley has been recommended for children who present with trigger thumb after 1 year of age, who fail conservative management, or who manifest rigid deformity.[95] McAdams and colleagues[110] presented long-term results on 30 thumbs in 21 patients with an average follow-up of 15 years. They had no cases of recurrence and no functional deficits; 23% had slightly diminished IPJ motion and 18% had MPJ hyperextension. Abnormal motion was not associated with age at time of surgery. Children who had a longitudinal incision had some concerns regarding scar appearance, and they thus recommended a transverse skin incision.

Recently, there has been some discussion regarding the anatomy of the thumb pulley system and how it may play a role in the pathophysiology of the trigger thumb. Doyle and Blythe described the anatomy of the thumb in 1977 as consisting of two annular pulleys (A1 and A2) with one oblique pulley.[111] They concluded that the oblique pulley was important for normal flexor pollicis longus tendon function and noted decreasing IPJ motion

and increasing MPJ motion as pulleys were sectioned. In biomechanical studies, Zissimos and colleagues[112] and Esplin and colleagues[113] determined that either an intact A1 or oblique pulley was necessary for normal kinematics.

Several researchers have noted additional structures, however. Bayat and colleagues[114] noted a distinct annular pulley between A1 and the oblique pulley, which they called the variable annular pulley (Av) and concluded that the oblique pulley did not play a role in the prevention of bowstringing of the flexor pollicis longus. They found that either the A1 or the Av pulley needed to remain intact for normal function. Considerable variation was noted in the anatomy of this pulley, but in its oblique form it was noted to run from proximal ulnar to distal radial.

In contrast to most authors who have recommended division of the A1 pulley[110,115] for the treatment of pediatric trigger thumb, van Loveren[116] determined that this was sufficient to resolve the triggering in only 3 out of 19 thumbs. It was necessary to release an additional structure found distal to the A1 pulley in 69% of cases. In two cases, a completely distinct additional annular pulley structure distal to the A1 pulley was identified and resection of this alone resolved the triggering.

They cautioned that the A1 pulley may not be the main or even causative structure involved in pediatric trigger thumb.

Boretto and colleagues[117] recently performed a prospective clinical study of the A1 pulley in 19 adult trigger thumbs. In 7 thumbs, they found pulleys with a combination of annular and oblique fibers that mimicked those described by Bayat and colleagues[114] as the A1 and the Av pulleys. In contrast to these authors, however, they did not believe that this represented a discrete separate structure. In contrast to van Loveren, sectioning of the standard A1 pulley was sufficient to resolve triggering in the majority (12 of 19) of patients.[110,116] This finding may represent differences in the pediatric and adult populations.

It is unclear whether the Av pulley as described by Bayat, the unnamed additional structure and separate annular pulley as described by van Loveren, and the A1 pulley with combined annular and oblique fibers as noted by Boretto represent the same structure.[114,116,117] It is possible that variants in pulley anatomy may contribute to pediatric trigger thumb. Variations in the pulley system and differences in which structures are sectioned may account for changes in range of motion after trigger thumb surgery.

REFERENCES

1. Mennen U, Van Heest A, Ezaki M, et al. Arthrogryposis multiplex congenital. J Hand Surg [Br] 2005;30(5):468–74.
2. Hall JG. Arthrogryposis. Am Fam Physician 1989;39(1):113–9.
3. Stern WG. Arthrogryposis multiplex congenita. JAMA 1923;81:1507–10.
4. Sheldon W. Amyoplasia congenital. Arch Dis Child 1932;7:117–36.
5. Hall JG, Reed SD, Green G. The distal arthrogryposes: delineation of new entities—review and nosologic discussion. Am J Med Genet 1982;11(2):185–239.
6. Bamshad M, Jorde LB, Carey JC. A revised and extended classification of the distal arthrogryposis. Am J Med Genet 1996;65(4):277–81.
7. Beals RK. The distal arthrogryposes: a new classification of peripheral contractures. Clin Orthop Relat Res 2005;(435):203–10.
8. Sells JM, Jaffer KM, Hall JG. Amyoplasia, the most common type of arthrogryposis: the potential for good outcome. Pediatrics 1996;97(2):225–31.
9. Bernstein RM. Arthrogryposis and amyoplasia. J Am Acad Orthop Surg 2002;10(6):417–24.
10. Sarwark JF, MacEwen GD, Scott CI Jr. Amyoplasia (a common form of arthrogryposis). J Bone Joint Surg Am 1990;72(3):465–9.
11. Hall JG, Reed SD, Driscoll EP. Part I. Amyoplasia: a common, sporadic condition with congenital contractures. Am J Med Genet 1983;15(4):571–90.
12. Hall JG. Arthrogryposis multiplex congenita: etiology, genetics, classification, diagnostic approach, and general aspects. J Pediatr Orthop B 1997;6(3):159–66.
13. Hall JG, Reed SD, McGillivray BC, et al. Part II. Amyoplasia: twinning in amyoplasia—a specific type of arthrogryposis with an apparent excess of discordantly affected identical twins. Am J Med Genet 1983;15(4):591–9.
14. Clarren SK, Hall JG. Neuropathologic findings in the spinal cords of 10 infants with arthrogryposis. J Neurol Sci 1983;58(1):89–102.
15. Drachman DB, Banker BQ. Arthrogryposis multiplex congenital case due to disease of the anterior horn cells. Arch Neurol 1961;5:77–93.
16. Fahy MJ, Hall JG. A retrospective study of pregnancy complications among 828 cases of arthrogryposis. Genet Couns 1990;1(1):3–11.
17. Ezaki M. Treatment of the upper limb in the child with arthrogryposis. Hand Clin 2000;16(4):703–11.
18. Bevan WP, Hall JG, Bamshad M. Arthrogryposis multiplex congenita (amyoplasia): an orthopaedic perspective. J Pediatr Orthop 2007;27(5):594–600.
19. Van Heest A, Waters PM, Simmons BP. Surgical treatment of arthrogryposis of the elbow. J Hand Surg [Am] 1998;23(6):1063–70.
20. Van Heest A, James MA, Lewica A, et al. Posterior elbow capsulotomy with triceps lengthening for treatment of elbow extension contracture in children with arthrogryposis. J Bone Joint Surg Am 2008;90(7):1517–23.
21. Kroksmark AK, Kimber E, Jerre R, et al. Muscle involvement and motor function in amyoplasia. Am J Med Genet A 2006;140(16):1757–67.
22. Smith DW, Drennan JC. Arthrogryposis wrist deformities: results of infantile serial casting. J Pediatr Orthop 2002;22(1):44–7.
23. Mennen U. Early corrective surgery of the wrist and elbow in arthrogryposis multiplex congenital. J Hand Surg [Br] 1993;18(3):304–7.
24. Goldfarb CA, Burke MS, Strecker WB, et al. The Steindler flexorplasty for the arthrogrypotic elbow. J Hand Surg [Am] 2004;29(3):462–9.
25. Wenner SM, Saperia BS. Proximal row carpectomy in arthrogrypotic wrist deformity. J Hand Surg [Am] 1987;12(4):523–5.
26. Weeks P. Surgical correction of upper extremity deformities in arthrogrypotics. Plast Reconstr Surg 1965;36(4):459–65.
27. Williams PF. Management of upper limb problems in arthrogryposis. Clin Ortho Relat Res 1985;194:60–7.
28. Ezaki M, Carter PR. Carpal wedge osteotomy for the arthrogrypotic wrist. Tech Hand Up Extrem Surg 2004;8(4):224–8.

29. Smith RJ, Kaplan EB. Camptodactyly and similar atraumatic flexion deformities of the proximal interphalangeal joints of the fingers: a study of thirty-one cases. J Bone Joint Surg Am 1968;50(6):1187–203.

30. Jones KG, Marmor L, Lankford LL. An overview on new procedures in surgery of the hand. Clin Orthop Relat Res 1974;99:154–67.

31. Benson LS, Waters PM, Kamil NI, et al. Camptodactyly: classification and results of nonoperative treatment. J Pediatr Orthop 1994;14(6):814–9.

32. Welch JP, Temtamy SA. Hereditary contractures of the fingers (camptodactyly). J Med Genet 1966; 3(2):104–13.

33. Koman LA, Toby EB, Poehling GG. Congenital flexion deformities of the proximal interphalangeal joint in children: a subgroup of camptodactyly. J Hand Surg [Am] 1990;15(4):582–6.

34. Gupta A, Burke FD. Correction of camptodactyly: preliminary results of extensor indicis transfer. J Hand Surg [Br] 1990;15(2):168–70.

35. Millesi H. Camptodactyly. In: Littler JW, Cramer LM, Smith JW, editors. Symposium on reconstructive hand surgery. St Louis (MO): CV Mosby; 1974. p. 175–7.

36. McFarlane RM, Curry GI, Evans HB. Anomalies of the intrinsic muscles in camptodactyly. J Hand Surg [Am] 1983;8(5 Pt 1):531–44.

37. Ogino T, Kato H. Operative findings in camptodactyly of the little finger. J Hand Surg [Br] 1992;17(6):661–4.

38. McCash CR. Congenital contractures of the hand. In: Stack HG, Bolton H, editors. The proceedings of the second hand club. London: British Society for Surgery of the Hand; 1970. p. 399–401.

39. Miura T. Non-traumatic flexion deformity of the proximal interphalangeal joint—its pathogenesis and treatment. Hand 1983;15(1):25–34.

40. Todd AH. A case of hereditary contracture of the little fingers (kamptodactyly). Lancet 1929;2:1088–9.

41. Smith PJ, Grobbelaar AO. Camptodactyly: a unifying theory and approach to surgical treatment. J Hand Surg [Am] 1998;23(1):14–9.

42. Hori M, Nakamura R, Inoue G, et al. Nonoperative treatment of camptodactyly. J Hand Surg [Am] 1987;12(6):1061–5.

43. McFarlane RM, Classen DA, Porte AM, et al. The anatomy and treatment of camptodactyly of the small finger. J Hand Surg [Am] 1992;17(1):35–44.

44. Siegert JJ, Cooney WP, Dobyns JH. Management of simple camptodactyly. J Hand Surg [Br] 1990; 15(2):181–9.

45. Lecercq C, Moneta MR. The treatment of congenital clinodactyly of the hand. Ital J Orthop Traumatol 1989;15(3):339–42.

46. Skvarilová B, Smahel Z. Clinodactyly—frequency and morphological implications. Acta Chir Plast 1984;26(2):72–8.

47. Hersh AH, Demarinis F, Stecher RM. On the inheritance and development of clinodactyly. Am J Hum Genet 1953;5:257–68.

48. Flatt AE. The care of congenital hand anomalies. 2nd edition. St. Louis (MO): Quality Medical Publishing, Inc.; 1994. p. 207.

49. Al-Qattan MM. Congenital sporadic clinodactyly of the index finger. Ann Plast Surg 2007;59(6):682–7.

50. Burke F, Flatt A. Clinodactyly: a review of a series of cases. Hand 1979;11(3):269–80.

51. Jones GB. Delta phalanx. J Bone Joint Surg Br 1964;46:226–8.

52. Light TR, Odgen JA. The longitudinal epiphyseal bracket: implications for surgical correction. J Pediatr Orthop 1981;1(3):299–305.

53. Vickers D. Clinodactyly of the little finger: a simple operative technique for reversal of the growth abnormality. J Hand Surg [Br] 1987;12B:335–42.

54. Caouette-Laberge L, Laberge C, Egerszeki EP, et al. Physiolysis for correction of clinodactyly in children. J Hand Surg [Am] 2002;27(4):659–65.

55. Smith RJ. Osteotomy for the "delta-phalanx" deformity. Clin Orthop 1977;123:91–4.

56. Evans DM, James NK. A bipedicled neurovascular step-advancement flap for soft tissue lengthening in clinodactyly. Br J Plast Surg 1992;45(5):380–4.

57. Arora AS, Chung KC, Otto W. Madelung and the recognition of Madelung's deformity. J Hand Surg [Am] 2006;31(2):177–82.

58. Zebala LP, Manske PR, Goldfarb CA. Madelung's deformity: a spectrum of presentation. J Hand Surg [Am] 2007;32(9):1393–401.

59. De Smet L, Claessens A, Fabry G. Gymnast wrist. Acta Orthop Belg 1993;59(4):377–80.

60. Herdman RC, Langer LO, Good RA. Dyschondrosteosis: the most common cause of Madelung's deformity. J Pediatr 1966;68(3):432–41.

61. Plafki C, Luetke A, Willbuerger RE, et al. Bilateral Madelung's deformity without signs of dyschondrosteosis within five generations in a European family—case report and review of the literature. Arch Orthop Trauma Surg 2000;120(1-2):114–7.

62. Belin V, Cusin V, Viot G, et al. SHOX mutations in dyschondrosteosis (Leri-Weill syndrome). Nat Genet 1998;19(1):67–9.

63. Shears DJ, Vassal HJ, Goodman FR, et al. Mutation and deletion of the pseudoautosomal gene SHOX cause Leri-Weill dyschondrosteosis. Nat Genet 1998;19(1):70–3.

64. Ross JL, Scott C Jr, Marttila P, et al. Phenotypes associated with SHOX deficiency. J Clin Endocrinol Metab 2001;86(12):5674–80.

65. Lippe B. Turner syndrome. Endocrinol Metab Clin North Am 1991;20(1):121–52.

66. Munns CF, Glass IA, LaBrom R, et al. Histopathological analysis of Leri-Weill dyschondrosteosis: disordered growth plate. Hand Surg 2001;6(1):13–23.

67. Marchini A, Marttila T, Winter A, et al. The short stature homeodomain protein SHOX induces cellular growth arrest and apoptosis and is expressed in human growth plate chondrocytes. J Biol Chem 2004;279(35):37103–14.

68. Vickers D, Nielsen G. Madelung deformity: surgical prophylaxis (physiolysis) during the late growth period by resection of the dyschondrosteosis lesion. J Hand Surg [Br] 1992;17(4):401–7.

69. Carter PR, Ezaki M. Madelung's deformity: surgical correction through the anterior approach. Hand Clin 2000;16(4):713–21.

70. Murphy MS, Linscheid RL, Dobyns JH, et al. Radial opening wedge osteotomy in Madelung's deformity. J Hand Surg [Am] 1996;21(6):1035–44.

71. Dannenberg M, Anton JI, Spiegel MB. Madelung's deformity (consideration of its roentgenological diagnostic criteria). Am J Roentgenol 1939;42: 671–6.

72. Salon A, Serra M, Pouliquen JC. Long-term follow-up of surgical correction of Madelung's deformity with conservation of the distal radioulnar joint in teenagers. J Hand Surg [Br] 2000;25(1):22–5.

73. dos Reis FB, Katchburian MV, Faloppa F, et al. Osteotomy of the radius and ulna for the Madelung deformity. J Bone Joint Surg Br 1998;80(5):817–24.

74. McCarroll HR, James MA, Newmeyer WL, et al. Madelung's deformity: quantitative assessment of x-ray deformity. J Hand Surg [Am] 2005;30(6):1211–20.

75. Tuder D, Frome B, Green DP. Radiographic spectrum of severity in Madelung's deformity. J Hand Surg [Am] 2008;33(6):900–4.

76. McCarroll HR, James MA, Newmeyer WL, et al. Madelung's deformity: quantitative radiographic comparison with normal wrists. J Hand Surg [Br] 2008;33(5):632–5.

77. James MA, Bednar M. Deformities of the wrist and forearm. In: Green DP, Hotchkiss RN, Pederson WC, et al, editors. Green's operative hand surgery. 5th edition. Philadelphia: Elsevier; 2005. p. 1469–506.

78. Fagg PS. Wrist pain in the Madelung's deformity of dyschondrosteosis. J Hand Surg [Br] 1988;13(1): 11–5.

79. Bruno RJ, Blank JE, Ruby LK, et al. Treatment of Madelung's deformity in adults by ulna reduction osteotomy. J Hand Surg [Am] 2003;28(3):421–6.

80. Harley BJ, Carter PR, Ezaki M. Volar surgical correction of Madelung's deformity. Tech Hand Up Extrem Surg 2002;6(1):30–5.

81. Harley BJ, Brown C, Cummings K, et al. Volar ligament release and distal radius dome osteotomy for correction of Madelung's deformity. J Hand Surg 2006;31A:1499–506.

82. Ranawat CS, DeFiore J, Straub LR. Madelung's deformity. an end-result study of surgical treatment. J Bone Joint Surg Am 1975;57(6):772–5.

83. Glard Y, Gay A, Launay F, et al. Isolated wedge osteotomy of the ulna for mild Madelung's deformity. J Hand Surg [Am] 2007;32(7):1037–42.

84. de Paula EJ, Cho AB, Mattar R, et al. Madelung's deformity: treatment with radial osteotomy and insertion of a trapezoidal wedge. J Hand Surg [Am] 2006;31(7):1206–13.

85. Houshian S, Schrøder HA, Weeth R. Correction of Madelung's deformity by the Ilizarov technique. J Bone Joint Surg Br 2004;86(4):536–40.

86. Schroven I, De Smet L, Zachee B, et al. Radial osteotomy and Sauvé-Kapandji procedure for deformities of the distal radius. Acta Orthop Belg 1995; 61(1):1–5.

87. White G, Weiland A. Madelung's deformity: treatment by osteotomy of the radius and Lauenstein procedure. J Hand Surg [Am] 1987;12(2):202–4.

88. Potenza V, Farsetti P, Caterini R. Isolated Madelung's deformity: long-term follow-up study of five patients treated surgically. J Pediatr Orthop B 2007;16(5):331–5.

89. Cardon LM, Ezaki M, Carter PR. Trigger finger in children. J Hand Surg [Am] 1999;24(6):1156–61.

90. Bae DS, Sodha S, Waters PM. Surgical treatment of the pediatric trigger finger. J Hand Surg [Am] 2007; 32(7):1043–7.

91. Van Heest AE, House J, Krivit W, et al. Surgical treatment of carpal tunnel syndrome and trigger digits in children with mucopolysaccharide storage disorders. J Hand Surg [Am] 1998;23(2):236–43.

92. Hirata H, Fujisawa K, Sasaki H, et al. Congenital trigger of the index finger at the A2 pulley. J Hand Surg [Br] 1996;21(5):609–11.

93. Tordai P, Engkvist O. Trigger fingers in children. J Hand Surg [Am] 1999;24(6):1162–5.

94. Bae DS. Pediatric trigger thumb. J Hand Surg [Am] 2008;33(7):1189–91.

95. Dinham JM, Meggitt BF. Trigger thumbs in children. A review of the natural history and indications for treatment in 105 patients. J Bone Joint Surg Br 1974;56(1):153–5.

96. Rodgers WB, Waters PM. Incidence of trigger digits in newborns. J Hand Surg [Am] 1994;19(3):364–8.

97. Slakey JB, Henrrickus WL. Acquired thumb flexion contracture in children: congenital trigger thumb. J Bone Joint Surg Br 1996;78(3):481–3.

98. Kikuchi N, Ogino T. Incidence and development of trigger thumb in children. J Hand Surg [Am] 2006; 31(4):541–3.

99. Notta A. Recherches sur affection particuliere des gaines tendineuses de la main, caracterisee par le developpement d'une nodosite sur le trajet des tendons flechisseurs des doigts et par l'empechement de leurs mouvements. [Research on a particular lesion of the tendon of the hand characterized by development of a nodule on the flexor tendon of the finger interfering with movement]. Archives

Générales de Medicine. Arch Med Gen Trop 1850; 24:142–61 [in French].

100. Fahey JJ, Bollinger JA. Trigger-finger in adults and children. J Bone Joint Surg Am 1954;36(6): 1200–18.

101. Ogino T. Trigger thumb in children: current recommendations for treatment. J Hand Surg [Am] 2008; 33(6):982–4.

102. Sugimoto Y, Matsui T, Inoue H, et al. [Long-term follow-up of snapping finger in children]. Seikeigeka (Orthop Surg) 1981;32:1726–31 [in Japanese].

103. Specher EE. Trigger thumbs in infants. J Bone Joint Surg Am 1949;31(3):672–4.

104. Buchman MT, Gibson TW, McCallum D, et al. Transmission electron microscopic pathoanatomy of congenital trigger thumb. J Pediatr Orthop 1999;19(3):411–2.

105. Neu BR, Murray JF. Congenital bilateral trigger digits in twins. J Hand Surg [Am] 1983;8(3):350–2.

106. Shim VC, Admire AA, Reidenreich RA, et al. Autosomal dominant inheritance pattern for trigger thumb. Plast Reconstr Surg 2002;109(1):240–1.

107. Baek GH, Kim JH, Chung MS, et al. The natural history of pediatric trigger thumb. J Bone Joint Surg Am 2008;90(5):980–5.

108. Watanbe H, Hamada Y, Toshima T, et al. Conservative treatment for trigger thumb in children. Arch Orthop Trauma Surg 2001;121(7):388–90.

109. Lee ZL, Chang CH, Yand WY, et al. Extension splint for trigger thumb in children. J Pediatr Orthop 2006;26(6):785–7.

110. McAdams TR, Moneim MS, Omer GE. Long-term follow-up of surgical release of the A1 pulley in childhood trigger thumb. J Pediatr Orthop 2002;22:41–3.

111. Dolye JR, Blythe WF. Anatomy of the flexor tendon sheath and pulleys of the thumb. J Hand Surg [Am] 1977;2(2):149–51.

112. Zissimos AG, Szabo RM, Yinger KE, et al. Biomechanics of the thumb flexor pulley system. J Hand Surg [Am] 1994;19(3):475–9.

113. Esplin VS, Tencer AF, Hanel DP, et al. Restoration of function of the thumb flexor apparatus requires repair of the oblique and one adjacent flexor tendon pulley. J Orthop Res 1996;14(1):152–6.

114. Bayat A, Shaaban H, Giakas G, et al. The pulley system of the thumb: anatomic and biomechanical study. J Hand Surg [Am] 2002;27(4):628–35.

115. Ger E, Kupcha P, Ger D. The management of trigger thumb in children. J Hand Surg [Am] 1991;16(5):944–7.

116. van Loveren, van der Biezen JJ. The congenital trigger thumb: is release of the first annular pulley alone sufficient to resolve the triggering? Ann Plast Surg 2007;58(3):335–7.

117. Boretto J, Alfie V, Donndorff A, et al. A prospective clinical study of the A1 pulley in trigger thumbs. J Hand Surg Eur Vol 2008;33(3):260–5.

Duplication

Andrew J. Watt, MD[a], Kevin C. Chung, MD[b],*

KEYWORDS

- Congenital • Duplication • Polydactyly
- Thumb duplication • Mirror hand

Congenital anomalies of the upper extremity present a formidable aesthetic and functional challenge for the reconstructive surgeon. Over the past half-century, surgeons and scientists have begun not only to characterize these anatomical aberrations but also to elucidate the underlying embryologic mechanisms responsible for these deformities. Congenital deformities affect 1% to 2% of all newborns, and 10% of these deformities involve the upper extremity.[1,2]

Congenital limb anomalies are classified according to the embryonic failure that underlies their clinical presentations. The most widely accepted classification, proposed by Frantz and O'Rahilly and modified by Swanson, divides these anomalies into seven categories of embryologic failure: failure of formation of parts, failure of differentiation, duplication, overgrowth, undergrowth, congenital constriction band syndrome, and generalized skeletal abnormalities.[3,4] This article addresses Swanson's category of duplication, inclusive of pre- and post-axial polydactyly, central polydactyly, and mirror hand, and provides a review of the relevant embryology, anatomy, surgical approach, and outcomes of intervention.

EMBRYOLOGY AND MOLECULAR MECHANISMS

Upper extremity development begins after 4 weeks of gestation and culminates in a functionally complex, anatomically mature limb by 8 weeks of gestation. The majority of congenital anomalies occur during this 4-week period of rapid limb development. Embryologic development happens in a highly orchestrated temporal and spatial fashion by relying on interactions among three known signaling centers and a host of transcription factors, secreted proteins, and receptors. The three primary signaling centers consist of the apical ectodermal ridge (AER), the zone of polarizing activity (ZPA), and the Wingless-type signaling center (WNT).

The AER is a specialized region of the ectoderm that condenses over the developing limb bud and mediates proximal to distal orientation. The AER specifically expresses a number of signaling molecules in the fibroblast growth factor family (FGF-2, -4, -8) that coordinate growth along the proximal-to-distal axis and is responsible for interdigital apoptosis.[5,6] Although the AER supplies these factors, there is clearly a complex interaction with the underlying mesoderm.

The ZPA exists within the lateral plate mesoderm and its position is determined prior to the formation of the limb bud itself. The ZPA determines the anterior-to-posterior (radio-ulnar) axis via secretion of the sonic hedgehog (SHH) protein.[5,7] In addition to this critical role in determining radio-ulnar growth, SHH is also necessary for the maintenance of proximal-to-distal growth by inducing FGF-4 expression in the AER.[8,9] This interrelationship dictates proportional growth along these two axes. Misplacement of this signaling center or aberrant production of SHH results in duplication of elements along the radio-ulnar axis and provides a plausible pathway in congenital errors of duplication.[6,10]

The WNT signaling center resides in the dorsal ectoderm and secretes WNT-7a, which defines the dorsal differentiation pathway.[7]

Supported in part by a Midcareer Investigator Award in Patient-Oriented Research (K24AR053120) from the National Institute of Arthritis and Musculoskeletal and Skin Diseases.

[a] Division of Plastic and Reconstructive Surgery, Department of Surgery, Stanford University Hospitals and Clinics, 770 Welch Road, Suite 400, Palo Alto, CA 94304, USA

[b] Section of Plastic Surgery, Department of Surgery, University of Michigan Medical School, 2130 Taubman Center, 1500 E. Medical Center Drive, Ann Arbor, MI 48109-0340, USA

* Corresponding author.

E-mail address: kecchung@umich.edu (K.C. Chung).

A complementary protein, engrailed-1, exists in the ventral portion of the limb. As the limb develops along these three axes, a series of Homeobox (HOX) genes are expressed in specific regions of the limb and are responsible for the ultimate differentiation of the highly specialized tissues of the upper extremity.[11–14] At this time, the exact molecular signals that activate these HOX genes remain unclear; however, signaling molecules including SHH have been implicated.

The exact molecular mechanisms that are responsible for congenital duplications of the hand are likely heterogenous; however, several chromosomal loci have shown a clear association with polydactyly. Polydactyly is a clinical characteristic of 119 phenotypic disorders and has been associated with 39 genetic mutations.[15] The most clearly defined are several examples of SHH misregulation resulting in pre-axial polydactyly. Several investigators have defined mutations in a ZPA regulatory sequence (ZRS).[16,17] This sequence has been mapped to the long arm of chromosome 7 and is highly conserved throughout a variety of species. The ZRS appears to act as a CIS-regulatory element controlling the expression of SHH. Single base-pair substitutions have been associated with pre-axial polydactyly, triphalangeal thumb, and triphalangeal thumb-polysyndactyly.[18–20] It is clear that with time, molecular research will continue to define more specific loci and genetic mechanisms responsible for disorders of duplication.

PRE-AXIAL POLYDACTYLY

Pre-axial polydactyly encompasses a range of congenital anomalies of the thumb. Thumb polydactyly or duplication is the second most common congenital hand disorder, and the incidence of pre-axial polydactyly is reported as 1 in every 3,000 live births.[21] Duplication alone is typically unilateral and sporadic; however, duplication in the setting of a triphalangeal thumb is inherited in an autosomal dominant pattern. Polydactyly of the thumb ranges from a vestigial radial skin tag to varying degrees of splitting to complete duplication. Depending on the level of duplication, anatomic variation presents a complexity of challenges.

Classification

Thumb duplications are classified according to the level of duplication. Wassel's classification is the most widely accepted and applied; however, several investigators have proposed a variety of subclasses for Type IV as well as triphalangeal thumbs.[22] Wassel's classification is based distal to proximal. Uneven numbers refer to bifid or incomplete duplications. Even numbers refer to complete duplications and Type VII refers to duplications with triphalangism (**Table 1**). This classification scheme is simple, descriptive, and clinically relevant; however, as several investigators have noted, the Wassel classification does not fully describe the anatomic complexity that is associated with thumb duplication. Type IV thumbs may be subdivided into subtypes A, B, and C, each of which contains a triphalangeal component. Type IV A is characterized by duplication at the level of the proximal phalanx, with two triphalanageal components articulating with a common metacarpal head. Types IV B and C are characterized by duplication at the level of the proximal phalanx with a single triphalangeal component arising on the radial and ulnar sides respectively.[23,24] Wood also further subdivided Wassel's triphalangism designation into four subtypes: *A*, in which the triphalangeal ray originates at the level of the metacarpal on the ulnar side; *B*, in which a radial and an ulnar triphalangeal ray originate at the level of the metacarpal; *C*, in which the triphalangeal ray originates at the level of the metacarpal on the radial side; and *D*, in which a central triphalangeal ray articulates with hypoplastic, nontriphalangeal rays on either side (triplication).[23]

Recently, Zuidam and colleagues[25] have proposed an adjusted nomenclature that allows classification of triphalangeal components and triplication in radial polydactyly. Zuidam's classification assigns roman numerals in a distal-to-proximal system analogous to Wassel's classification. Type VII refers to a bifid trapezium. Type VIII refers to a duplicated trapezium. Abbreviations for triphalangism (Tph), triplication (T), symphalangism (S), deviation (D), and hypoplasia (H) are introduced. The position of the duplicated part is assigned according to the ulnar (u), middle (m), or radial (r) position. Triplication is classified by first assigning the most proximal duplication, followed by the distal duplication. For example, duplication at the level of the proximal phalanx with a triphalangeal component on the ulnar aspect, is classified as Type IV Tph u.

Anatomy

The complexity of classification in pre-axial polydactyly suggests that the pathologic anatomy is both variable and complex. The recognition that none of the anatomic components of either duplicate are normal is paramount. The surgeon must also consider the level of duplication, the degree of hypoplasia of each component, stability of the involved joints, and position of the thumb with respect to the bony axis and first web space.

Table 1
Classification of thumb duplication

Wassel Type	Anatomic Description	%	
Type I	Bifid Distal Phalanx	4%	
Type II	Duplicated Distal Phalanx sharing common Distal Interphalangeal Joint articulation	16%	
Type III	Bifid Proximal Phalanx	11%	
Type IV	Duplicated Proximal Phalanx sharing common Metacarpal articulation	40%	
Type V	Bifid Metacarpal	10%	
Type VI	Duplicated Metacarpal sharing common Carpal articulation	4%	
Type VII	Triphalangeal Thumb	20%	

Data from Wassel HD. The results of surgery for polydactyly of the thumb. Clin Orthop Relat Res 1969;64:175–93; and Townsend DJ, Lipp EB, Chun K, et al. Thumb duplication, 66 years experience: a review of surgical complications. J Hand Surg [Am] 1994;19(6):973–6.

The osseous anatomy is abnormal, with varying degrees of bony hypoplasia as well as widening and angulation of the articular surfaces. The flexor and extensor tendons are split and insert eccentrically.[26] An abnormal connection between the flexor and extensor tendons on the radial aspect of the thumb often exists as well. The origins and insertions of the thenar musculature, particularly the opponens pollicis, are aberrant in cases of proximal duplication.[27] The abductor pollicis brevis (APB) and flexor pollicis brevis (FPB) insert into the proximal phalanx of the radial-most duplicate while the opponens pollicis inserts into the radial metacarpal. The net effect of the long flexor tendons is to pull the distal phalanges into convergence while the thenar insertions create divergence at the proximal phalangeal level, creating a zig-zag deformity (**Fig. 1**). Finally, the arterial supply of the duplicated thumb most commonly consists of single digital arteries located on the ulnar side of the ulnar and radial duplicates. This arterial supply is present in 74% of cases. Twelve percent of patients exhibit three digital arteries, located on the radial and ulnar sides of the ulnar duplicate and the ulnar side of the radial duplicate. Ten percent of patients exhibit four digital arteries and 5% maintain a single digital artery associated with the ulnar duplicate.[28]

Surgical Treatment

Surgical treatment for congenital thumb duplication has evolved from simple ablation of the hypoplastic duplicate to a concerted reconstruction utilizing the shared anatomic components. Initial descriptions of surgical intervention failed to recognize the anatomic complexity of reconstruction. In 1957, Kelikian and Doumanian stated "an extra finger or thumb is removed for cosmetic reasons. This operation requires no ingenuity and creates no problems."[29] Longitudinal studies, however, have demonstrated that ablation alone results in unacceptable thumb function and the need for revisional operations in 40% to 56% of cases.[30,31]

Reconstruction of the duplicated thumb ideally seeks to restore or approximate normal anatomy via manipulation of the skeletal and soft-tissue elements in an effort to achieve a reasonable,

functional, and aesthetic outcome. Surgical options vary according to the level of duplication and the anatomy of the available tissue components. These operations include ablation with collateral ligament reconstruction, the Bilhaut procedure, and on-top plasty. The timing of operative intervention is dictated by the size of the available components, displacement of the ulnar thumb by the radial component, and by developmental considerations. Ideally the thumb should be of sufficient size to allow the anatomic components to be clearly defined and operation should occur prior to the development of significant deviation and the development of pinch grasp at 10 to 12 months. Generally, operative treatment occurs between 9 and 15 months of age.

Ablation with collateral ligament reconstruction

Surgical technique The technique of ablation with collateral ligament reconstruction is applicable to all types of thumb duplication. This operation is particularly well suited for Type IV and Type VI duplications in which a clearly more hypoplastic, less-functional thumb exists. Consideration is given to the relative size and function of the two thumbs. When possible, the ulnar thumb is preserved in an effort to maintain the ulnar collateral ligament, which is more difficult to reconstruct than its radial counterpart.

An elliptical or zig-zag incision is made at the base of the accessory thumb. Care is taken to preserve the radial collateral ligament and it is then detached in a distal to proximal fashion, preserving a periosteal sleeve.[32] In cases of Type IV duplication, the APB and FPB, which insert on the proximal phalanx of the radial thumb, are elevated from their insertion. Elevation of the APB and FPB may be performed separately or in continuity with the radial collateral ligament via

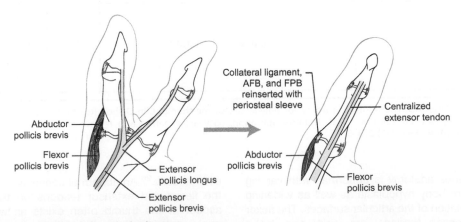

Fig. 1. Anatomy of Type IV thumb duplication.

the periosteum. The insertions of the extensor and flexor tendons for the radial digit are detached and elevated proximally for potential use to rebalance the ulnar thumb. The radial thumb is then amputated, while the soft-tissue elements necessary for reconstruction are preserved. The articular surface is examined and the articular cartilage is shaved or narrowed, if necessary. Because the phalanges are not ossified, bone removal can be performed with a sharp knife blade in a rocking motion. The distal elements are then centralized by fixation with a Kirschner wire and the radial collateral ligament with its periosteal sleeve is sutured to the radial side of the preserved ulnar thumb. The flexor and extensor tendons from the ablated radial thumb may be used to rebalance the ulnar thumb by suturing them to the distal phalanx (**Fig. 2**). Consideration is given to the opponens pollicis in cases of Type V and VI duplications. This muscle must be detached at its insertion into the metacarpal of the radial digit and transferred to the retained ulnar metacarpal.

In most instances, rebalancing of the soft tissue with collateral ligament reconstruction and tendon centralization corrects any angular deformity that may exist in the preserved thumb; however, cases exist in which osseous deformity disrupt the axial alignment of the thumb. In these cases, closing

or opening wedge osteotomies may be necessary to provide alignment. Bone graft is obtained from the amputated thumb.

Surgical outcomes Thumb reconstruction with ablation and collateral ligament reconstruction has several advantages. This technique preserves both the nail bed and physis, thereby preventing nail deformities and fostering normal axial growth over time. The reconstructed joints also tend to remain supple, without significant restriction in range of motion. Disadvantages include interphalangeal (IP) and metacarpophalangeal (MCP) joint instability, particularly against ulnarly directed forces, and size mismatch compared with the contralateral normal thumb. Naasan and Page[33] report secondary deformity, including joint laxity and unacceptable size mismatch in 4 out of 11 (36%) of cases treated by excision with collateral ligament reconstruction. Townsend and colleagues[31] report on 33 thumbs treated by ablation accompanied by a reconstructive procedure (collateral ligament reconstruction, tendon transfer/rerouting, osteotomy). In this series, 19 out of 33 (58%) thumbs were defined as acceptable, whereas 14 out of 33 (42%) were defined as unacceptable. Thumbs were defined as unacceptable if IP joint deviation or laxity

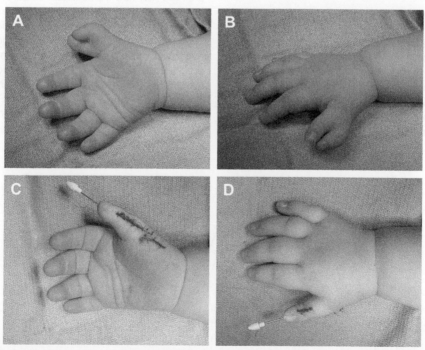

Fig. 2. Type IV thumb duplication. (*A*) Type IV thumb duplication preoperative, volar. (*B*) Type IV thumb duplication preoperative, dorsal. (*C*) Type IV thumb duplication postoperative, volar. (*D*) Type IV thumb duplication postoperative, dorsal.

exceeded 15°, MCP joint deviation or laxity exceeded 30°, and thumb size was one-third greater or less that the contralateral thumb or based on the examiner's overall assessment.

These results underscore the complexity of thumb reconstruction in cases of pre-axial polydactyly. The authors recommend ablation with collateral ligament reconstruction in all cases of thumb polydactyly in which a clearly hypoplastic duplicate exists. The authors routinely reconstruct the radial collateral ligament and use the remnant tendon from the excised radial thumb to rebalance the intact thumb. Wedge osteotomies are performed only if angular deformity persists after collateral ligament reconstruction and tendon rebalancing.

Bilhaut procedure

The technique of thumb reconstruction by combining the two hypoplastic thumb duplicates was first described in 1889 by Bilhaut.[34] This original description addresses Type I duplications; however, the technique has been adapted to address more proximal Wassel types.[35,36] This technique recognizes that neither duplicate thumb is anatomically normal, and is particularly well suited for Type I and II duplications (in which both thumbs are severely hypoplastic) and in markedly deviated thumbs (divergent at MCP, convergent at IP).

Surgical technique The Bilhaut technique is, in essence, a composite wedge resection of the central bone and soft-tissue components with approximation of the lateral tissue from each thumb. The nail bed may be split or retained in its entirety from one of the duplicates if its width is greater than 70% of the contralateral thumb.[37,38] In Types I and II, a V-shaped excision is designed. The duplicated distal phalanges are split via

longitudinal osteotomy, taking care to preserve the insertions of the flexor and extensor tendons. The bone is approximated, with attention paid to matching the physis and articular surface, and is secured with interosseous wires. The nail bed is then meticulously repaired (**Fig. 3**). Type III and IV duplications are approached via matching dorsal and volar zig-zag incisions. The extensor and flexor mechanisms are preserved and retracted laterally. Longitudinal osteotomies of the distal and proximal phalanges are performed. The phalanges are then approximated with attention paid to physeal and articular congruence. The tendon mechanisms are centralized and their insertions are explored if angulation exists.

Surgical outcomes The Bilhaut technique has several advantages. First, sufficient thumb size is typically obtained by combining two hypoplastic components. Second, the collateral ligaments are not violated during the reconstruction, resulting in very stable IP and MCP joints. Despite these advantages, several prominent disadvantages are inherent in the procedure. Violation of the physis, particularly across multiple joints, may result in growth arrest or asymmetric growth. Tonkin and Bulstrode emphasize the importance of exact physeal matching in an effort to avoid these complications.[39] Nail deformity is also common after repair and efforts should be made to utilize a single nail bed if possible. Although thumbs reconstructed with the Bilhaut technique have stable joints, they exhibit restricted flexion. Tonkin reports that IP flexion in a reconstructed thumb averaged 13°, compared with 68° in the contralateral thumb. MCP flexion in the reconstructed thumbs averaged 55°, compared with 75° in the contralateral thumb.[39] Naasan and Page report secondary deformities included growth abnormalities, joint stiffness, and nail bed deformities in

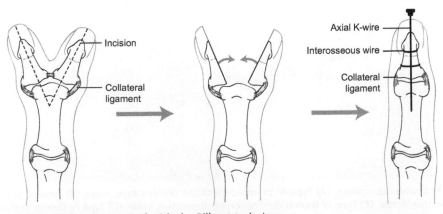

Fig. 3. Type II thumb duplication treated with the Bilhaut technique.

71% of the thumbs reconstructed with the Bilhaut technique.[33] Townsend and colleagues classified five out of five (100%) of thumbs treated with the Bilhaut technique as unacceptable.[31]

The authors may consider using the Bilhaut technique for cases of Type I and II duplication, and rarely for cases of Type III and IV duplication in which the duplicates are both markedly hypoplastic. Even with physeal matching and meticulous nail bed repair, the results are not satisfying.

On-top plasty procedure

The on-top plasty maintains a limited role in the treatment of congenital thumb duplication. This technique, initially described as a way to lengthen amputated digits, is applicable to duplications in which one thumb is larger proximally, while the other is larger distally. The goal is to combine the less-hypoplastic components to reconstruct a functional thumb. This technique is technically difficult and rarely employed in cases of thumb duplication.

Surgical technique The on-top plasty technique involves transferring the distal portion of a digit to an adjacent digit based on the neurovascular pedicle. In cases of thumb duplication, the less-hypoplastic distal component is transferred to the less-hypoplastic proximal component at the level of the mid-proximal phalanx or mid-metacarpal. The hypoplastic distal component is amputated, typically preserving the flexor and extensor tendons. A transverse osteotomy is made at the level of transfer (mid-proximal phalanx or mid-metacarpal). The component to be transferred is approached through a circumferential incision that may be extended proximally in a Y-fashion. Care is taken to identify and preserve the dominant neurovascular bundle radially or ulnarly. A transverse osteotomy is made and the distal component, supplied by its digital neurovascular bundle, is transferred through its arc of rotation to the proximal component. Osseous fixation is achieved via interosseous wiring or with Kirschner wire fixation. Eccentric flexor and extensor tendons are centralized and reinserted. Proximal duplications (Types IV, V, and VI) require reconstruction of the APB, FPB, and opponens pollicis as well.

Surgical outcomes No outcomes studies exist to evaluate the functional results of on-top plasty reconstruction. This procedure's utility in the reconstruction of pre-axial polydactyly is limited by its technical difficulty; however, the technique does offer the theoretical benefit of preserving the collateral ligaments, thus maintaining joint stability.

Secondary deformities

Long-term complications following reconstruction include diminished size, joint instability, and zig-zag or Z-deformity. These complications increase in frequency in direct relation to the complexity of the primary operation. Diminished size is best addressed at the time of the initial operation. The Bilhaut technique reliably provides sufficient tissue; however, the operation is plagued by issues of joint stiffness, nail deformity, and long-term growth complications. In contrast, ablation with collateral ligament reconstruction often results in a smaller thumb and joint laxity in 30% of cases.[33] Failure to recognize and correct eccentric insertion of the flexor and extensor tendons at the time of initial reconstruction results in chronic axial deviation or Z-deformity, which exacerbates articular change. Correction requires centralization and rebalancing of the tendons and, in cases with bony imbalance, corrective osteotomies to bring the thumb into axial alignment. In general, the Bilhaut technique is indicated in cases of Type I and II duplication and may be considered in cases of Type III or IV duplication when both components are markedly hypoplastic or exhibit significant divergence and convergence at the MCP and IP, respectively. Ablation with collateral ligament reconstruction is the preferred procedure in the remainder of congenital thumb duplications.

POST-AXIAL POLYDACTYLY

Post-axial polydactyly includes an array of congenital duplications involving the ulnar aspect of the hand. Unlike pre-axial polydactyly, which is distinctly more common in patients of European ancestry, post-axial polydactyly is more common in patients of African descent. The incidence is reported as 1 in 1,339 live births in Caucasians, compared with 1 in 143 live births in Africans and African Americans. The presence of post-axial polydactyly in patients of African ancestry is typically isolated, whereas in Caucasians it is often associated with an underlying syndrome.[40] Inheritance is most often autosomal dominant with incomplete penetrance; however, recessive inheritance has been reported, particularly in association with syndromic presentations.[41-46] Several isolated genetic defects have been definitively associated with ulnar polydactyly, including a frameshift mutation of the Gli3 gene on chromosome 7, and linkage to loci on the long arm of chromosome 13 and the short arm of chromosome 19.[45-47]

Anatomy and Classification

Phenotypic presentations of ulnar polydactyly range from a small skin appendage on the ulnar aspect of the hand to a fully formed ulnar digit articulating with a separate sixth metacarpal. Two classification schemes have been proposed. Stelling and Turek have classified ulnar polydactyly into three types: Type 1 consists of a floating appendage linked to the hand by a skin bridge, Type 2 encompasses partial duplication, and Type 3 refers to complete duplication of the metacarpal and phalanges.[48,49] More commonly, the classification of Temtamy and McKusick[50] is employed. This classification separates ulnar polydactyly into Type A, in which a well-formed duplicated digit articulates with the fifth or a sixth metacarpal, and Type B, in which a rudimentary, poorly developed ulnar duplication exists (**Table 2**).

Surgical Treatment

Type B polydactyly
Surgical technique Analogous to radial polydactyly, the level of duplication and anatomical components should guide operative treatment. Type B polydactyly is defined by the absence of osseous and ligamentous structures connecting the rudimentary digit to the hand (**Fig. 4**). Treatment, therefore, requires simple division of the skin bridge, which may be performed with surgical resection or, more commonly, suture ligation. Suture ligation is often performed by pediatricians in the newborn nursery. Ligation occludes the vascular supply to the duplicated digit, resulting in dry gangrene and subsequent autoamputation. Criticisms of suture ligation cite residual deformity, scarring, and infection. Although parents are concerned about accidental avulsion of the pedunculated digit, the senior author has not seen this happen. The authors' practice is not to ligate the digit, but rather perform excision in the operating room when the child is between 6 and 12 month of age.

Surgical outcomes Watson and Hennrikus[40] reported on 21 patients with Type B ulnar polydactyly treated with suture ligation. They found that the duplicated digit typically amputated at an average of 10 days and reported no complications of infection or bleeding. Rayan and Frey[51] reported on 105 patients treated with suture ligation. They document an overall complication rate of 23.5%, citing a residual tender or unacceptable bump in 16%, infection in 6%, and bleeding in 1% of patients. In general, suture ligation is safe and effective when applied to appropriate cases of Type B polydactyly in which no substantial ligamentous or osseous structures are present within the pedicle. Parents should be educated as to the progression of necrosis, and that revision of residual tissue or scar may be necessary when the child is 6 months of age or older.

Type A polydactyly
The treatment of Type A ulnar polydactyly is more complex and is, in many respects, analogous to the surgical treatment of radial polydactyly. The goal of surgical intervention is to remove the accessory digit while maintaining a stable, functional small finger. Consideration is given to the ulnar collateral ligament in cases where the duplicated proximal phalanx articulates with a common, broad metacarpal head; the abductor digiti minimi (ADM) must be preserved in cases of common articulation and in cases with a sixth metacarpal.

Surgical technique In Type A cases with a common metacarpal articulation, the post-axial digit is approached via an elliptical incision at its base. This incision may be extended proximally in order to adequately expose the ADM. The ulnar collateral ligament and ADM insertions are elevated with a periosteal sleeve. The duplicated extensor and flexor tendons to the postaxial digit are transected and the digit is amputated at its articulation with the metacarpal. The metacarpal may be shaved if the articular surface is wide and the collateral ligament and ADM are reinserted at the base of the preserved proximal phalanx. A Kirschner wire is then placed across the reconstructed joint (**Fig. 5**). In contrast to pre-axial polydactyly, the

---

Table 2
Classification of central polydactyly

Type	Anatomic Description
Type I	No osseous or ligamentous attachements, frequently devoid of bones, joints, cartilage or tendons
Type II	Normal components articulating with a broad or bifid metacarpal or phalanx. A: Nonsyndactylous B: Syndactylous
Type III	Complete digital duplication articulating with well-formed duplicated metacarpal

Data from Graham TJ, Ress AM. Finger polydactyly. Hand Clin 1998;14(1):49–64.

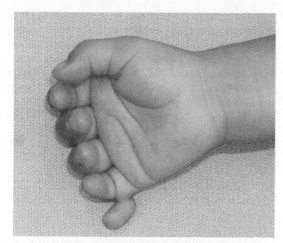

Fig. 4. Type B post-axial polydactyly.

retained small finger is relatively normal anatomically and typically is aligned in the proper axis; therefore, it is rare that the flexor or extensor tendons would require centralization or rerouting. In cases involving a duplicated metacarpal, the accessory digit is amputated in a standard ray fashion with transfer of the ADM to the retained small finger.

Surgical outcomes No substantive outcome studies exist regarding the function of these hands following surgical intervention. This lack of data is in large part because of the generally normal function of these patients' hands following ablation with collateral ligament reconstruction. Rayan and Frey reported on 27 patients undergoing surgical excision for Type A ulnar polydactyly, noting only one complication in the form of an infection.[51] No investigators have objectively reviewed functional range of motion or articular stability.

The authors recommend surgical excision with ligamentous reconstruction for Type A ulnar polydactyly between the age of 9 and 12 months. By this age, the anatomic components have reached sufficient size to allow for ease of identification and manipulation, and the risk of general anesthesia is reduced. The ADM insertion should be preserved and transferred via a periosteal sleeve to the retained duplicate along with the ulnar collateral ligament. The authors do not routinely explore the flexor or extensor tendons unless there is marked deviation of the retained digit to suggest eccentric insertion.

CENTRAL POLYDACTYLY

Central polydactyly includes duplications that occur within the hand and involve the index, middle, or ring fingers. Central polydactyly is uncommon when compared with thumb and ulnar duplication, and is often accompanied by

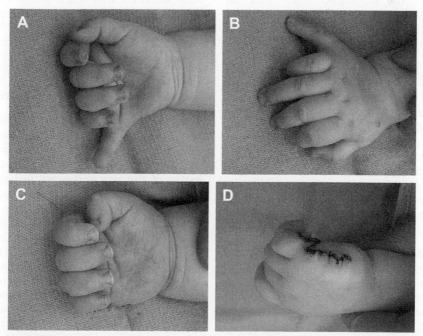

Fig. 5. Type A post-axial polydactyly. (*A*) Type A post-axial polydactyly pre-operative, volar. (*B*) Type A post-axial polydactyly pre-operative, dorsal. (*C*) Type A post-axial polydactyly post-operative, volar. (*D*) Type A post-axial polydactyly post-operative, dorsal.

syndactyly and cleft hand.[52,53] In his review of 144 cases of polydactyly at the University of Iowa, Wood[54] found 22 cases of central polydactyly. Over half of these patients had first-degree relatives with similar deformities, suggesting autosomal dominant inheritance. Of these 22 patients, 20 had an element of syndactyly or synpolydactyly. Tada and colleagues[53] reviewed 238 cases of polydactyly at the Osaka University Hospital, noting 12 cases of central polydactyly. Central polydactyly therefore includes a heterogenous group of duplications, which overlap with syndactyly (failure of differentiation of parts) and cleft hand (failure of formation of parts). Polysyndactyly of the ring finger has been linked to a mutation of the HoxD13 gene on chromosome 2.

Anatomy and Classification

Central polydactyly is classified into three types based on the extent of duplication. Type I refers to a central duplication that is not attached to the adjacent finger via osseous or ligamentous attachments and is frequently devoid of bones, joints, cartilage, or tendons. Type II includes a duplication of a digit or part of a digit that has normal components and articulates with a broad or bifid metacarpal or phalanx. This type is further subdivided into Type IIa (nonsyndactylous), and Type IIb (syndactylous). Type III consists of complete digital duplication, including a well-formed duplicated metacarpal.[52] The duplicated finger may be obvious in Types II or III or occult, hidden within the adjacent web space in cases of Type I and some Type II duplications.

Surgical Treatment

The surgical treatment of central polydactyly is highly variable and requires intraoperative creativity and flexibility in order to restore an aesthetically pleasing, functional and stable hand. The surgeon must also consider whether retention of a fully functional supranumerary digit is preferable to surgical intervention. In contrast, a functional, four-fingered hand achieved via ray amputation may be preferable to a five-fingered hand with a deformed or stiff reconstructed finger.

Surgical technique

Cases of polysyndactyly are approached through a standard opposing zig-zag incision. The incision is favored toward the accessory digit, preserving extra skin for subsequent closure. Depending on the level and extent of duplication, the flexor and extensor tendons may require centralization or rebalancing and the collateral ligaments must be preserved or reconstructed. Analogous to reconstruction of pre-axial polydactyly, wide articular surfaces should be narrowed and phalangeal wedge osteotomies may be required to provide for axial alignment. Attention must also be given to reconstruction of the intermetacarpal ligament and provision made for adequate web-space soft tissue.

Surgical outcomes

Few clinical outcome studies exist regarding the treatment of central polydactyly. Tada and colleagues[53] note that satisfactory surgical correction of central polydactyly is difficult to achieve and that outcomes are generally poor. In Tada's study, 12 patients were reviewed. All patients required secondary surgical procedures to address flexion contractures and angular deviation at the IP joint level. The investigators note several primary factors that contribute to the complexity of central polydactyly reconstruction, including hypoplastic joints and soft tissues that predispose the reconstructed finger to joint contracture, and angular deformities as well as complex tendon anomalies that are often difficult to address. The investigators ultimately suggest ray amputation with creation of a functional four-digit hand.

The treatment of central polydactyly is highly variable and is wholly dependent on the anatomic components present, the degree of syndactyly, and the function of the duplicated finger. The authors do not routinely address occult duplications within the web space unless they are functionally problematic. In general, the authors' preference is to reconstruct a functional, stable four- or five-digit hand based on the available components.

MIRROR HAND AND MULTIPLE-HAND SPECTRUM

Mirror hand is a pronounced example of duplication (**Table 3**). Mirror hand is an exceedingly rare deformity characterized by duplication of the ulna, absence of the radius and thumb, and duplication of the ring and small fingers about the midline defined by a common central finger. This deformity is further characterized by an absence of the extensor forearm musculature and a consequent flexion deformity of the wrist. Over time, the ulna will take on features of a radius; however, no distal radio-ulnar articulation is present and rotation at the level of the wrist is limited. Only six cases of true mirror hand, also referred to as ulnar dimelia, exist in the literature; however, a number of similar deformities are reported, ranging from mirror hand to multiple hand, in which two distinctly duplicated hands share a common, normal, forearm.[55,56]

Table 3
Classification of mirror hand/multiple hand spectrum

Type	Name	Clinical Presentation
Type 1	Ulnar dimelia	Ulna: duplicated Radius: absent Thumb: absent Fingers: multiple, duplicated about the midline
Type 2	Intermediate form	Ulna: duplicated Radius: present, hypoplastic Thumb: absent Fingers: multiple, duplicated about the midline
Type 3	Intermediate form	Ulna: single Radius: present, well formed (Type A), hypoplastic (Type B) Thumb: absent Fingers: multiple, duplicated about the midline
Type 4	Syndromic mirror hand	Bilateral, mirror feet, nasal defects Type A: Sandrow's syndrome Ulna: duplicated Radius: absent Thumb: absent Fingers: multiple, duplicated about the midline Type B: Martin's syndrome Ulna: single Radius: present Thumb: absent Fingers: multiple, duplicated about the midline
Type 5	Multiple hand	Ulna: single, normal Radius: single, normal Thumb: present, fully duplicated Fingers: present, fully duplicated

Data from Al-Qattan MM, Al-Thunayan A, De Cordier M, et al. Classification of the mirror hand-multiple hand spectrum. J Hand Surg [Br] 1998;23B(4):535.

This spectrum of abnormal development demonstrates a failure of antero-posterior differentiation and is plausibly associated with errors or duplications in the zone of polarizing activity or SHH expression. Saunders and Gasseling's early experiments in chick embryos, which established the role of the ZPA in defining the radio-ulnar axis, demonstrated mirror-type morphology when the ZPA was transplanted to the anterior margin of the developing limb bud.[57] Currently, no clear genetic anomalies or associations have been defined in human beings with mirror- or multiple-hand deformities.

Surgical treatment seeks to create a functional, aesthetic hand. This objective requires ablation of excess fingers and creation of a thumb via pollicization by transferring a digit on its neurovascular pedicle with shortening, transposition, and rotation of the transferred digit. The surgeon must decide which finger should be retained and which can be brought into the best functional position. Typically, the post-axial fingers are in better alignment, and the most normal pre-axial digit is pollicized by using the skin and soft tissues of the amputated fingers to create an adequate first web space. Wrist flexion contracture may be addressed with a combination of capsulotomy, excision of the proximal carpal row, or tendon transfer from the amputated digits to the preserved metacarpals.[58,59]

SUMMARY

Congenital duplications are complex functional and aesthetic problems. Our understanding of both the embryologic basis of these anomalies, as well as the anatomy underlying them, has greatly increased over the past 40 years. Surgical treatment has evolved from merely ablating the extra digit to involve careful consideration of the available components and ultimate functional outcome. Successful surgical intervention requires an appreciation of the level of duplication, availability, and quality of the duplicated components, as well as an understanding that these components are not normal, but rather hypoplastic to some degree. Reconstruction relies on ensuring proper axial alignment, centralization or rebalancing of eccentric tendons, and preservation of the collateral ligaments and associated musculature. An understanding of these fine technical considerations ensures a more functional and aesthetic reconstruction.

REFERENCES

1. Flatt AE. Extra thumbs. In: Flatt AE, editor. The care of congenital hand anomalies. St. Louis (MO): Mosby; 1977. p. 99–117.
2. McCarroll HR. Congenital anomalies: a 25-year overview. J Hand Surg [Am] 2000;25(6):1007–37.
3. Frantz CH, O'Rahilly R. Congenital skeletal limb deficiencies. J Bone Joint Surg Am 1961;43:1202–24.
4. Swanson AB. A classification for congenital limb malformations. J Hand Surg [Am] 1976;1:8–22.
5. Bamshad M, Watkins WS, Dixon ME, et al. Reconstructing the history of human limb development: lessons from birth defects. Pediatr Res 1999;45(3): 291–9.
6. Riddle RD, Tabin C. How limbs develop. Sci Am 1999;280(2):74–9.
7. Riddle RD, Ensini M, Nelson C, et al. Induction of the LIM Homeobox gene LMX1 by WNT7a establishes dorsoventral pattern in the vertebrate limb. Cell 1995;83:631–40.
8. Laufer E, Nelson CE, Johnson RL, et al. Sonic Hedgehog and FGF-4 act through a signaling cascade and feedback loop to integrate growth and patterning of the developing limb bud. Cell 1994;79(6):993–1003.
9. Niswander L, Tickle C, Vogel A, et al. Function of FGF-4 in limb development. Mol Reprod Dev 1994; 39(1):83–8.
10. Riddle RD, Johnson RL, Laufer E, et al. Sonic Hedgehog mediates the polarizing activity of the ZPA. Cell 1993;75:1401–16.
11. Mortlock DP, Post LC, Innis JW. The molecular basis of hypodactyly (Hd): a deletion in Hoxa 13 leads to arrest of digital arch formation. Nat Genet 1996; 13(3):284–9.
12. Nelson CW, Morgan BA, Burke AC, et al. Analysis of Hox gene expression in the chick limb bud. Development 1996;122(5):1449–66.
13. Tabin CJ. Retinoids, homeoboxes, and growth factors: toward molecular models for limb development. Cell 1991;66(2):199–217.
14. Zakany J, Fromental-Ramain C, Warot X, et al. Regulations of number and size of digits by posterior Hox genes: a dose-dependent mechanism with potenial evolutionary implications. Proc Natl Acad Sci U S A 1997;94(25):13695–700.
15. Biesecker LG. Polydactyly: how many disorders and how many genes. Am J Med Genet 2002;12(3):279–83.
16. Lettice LA, Hill LE, Devenney PS, et al. Point mutations in a distant sonic Hedgehog cis-regulator generate a variable regulatory output responsible for preaxial polydactyly. Hum Mol Genet 2008; 17(7):978–85.
17. Hill RE. How to make a zone of polarizing activity: insights into limb development via the abnormality preaxial polydactyly. Dev Growth Differ 2007;49(6): 439–48.
18. Heus HC, Hing A, van Baren MJ, et al. A physical and transcriptional map of the preaxial polydactyly locus on chromosome 7q36. Genomics 1999;57(3): 342–51.
19. Heutink P, Zguricas J, van Oosterhout L, et al. The gene for triphalangeal thumb maps to the subtelomeric region of chromosome 7q. Nat Genet 1994; 6(3):287–92.
20. Zguricas J, Heus H, Morales-Peralta E, et al. Clinical and genetic studies on 12 preaxial polydactyly families and refinement of the localisation of the gene responsible to a 1.9cM region on chromosome 7q36. J Med Genet 1999;36(1):32–40.
21. Jobe MT. Congenital anomalies of the hand. In: Canale ST, Beaty JH, editors. Campbell's operative orthopaedics. 11th edition. Philidelphia: Mosby; 2008. p. 4367–449.
22. Wassel HD. The results of surgery for polydactyly of the thumb. Clin Orthop Relat Res 1969;64:175–93.
23. Wood VE. Polydactyly and the triphalangeal thumb. J Hand Surg [Am] 1978;3(5):436–44.
24. Miura T. Triphalageal thumb. Plast Reconstr Surg 1976;58(5):587–94.
25. Zuidam JM, Selles RW, Ananata M, et al. A classification system of radial polydactyly: inclusion of triphalangeal thumb and triplication. J Hand Surg [Am] 2008;33:373–7.
26. Miura T. An appropriate treatment for postoperative Z-formed deformity of the duplicated thumb. J Hand Surg [Am] 1977;2(5):380–6.
27. Marks TW, Bayne LG. Polydactyly of the thumb: abnormal anatomy and treatment. J Hand Surg [Am] 1978;3(2):107–16.
28. Kitayama Y, Tsukada S. Patterns of arterial distribution in the duplicated thumb. Plast Reconstr Surg 1983;72(4):535–41.
29. Kelikian H, Doumanian A. Congenital anomalies of the hand, part I. J Bone Joint Surg Am 1957;39: 1002–19.
30. Miura T. Duplicated thumb. Plast Reconstr Surg 1982;69(3):470–81.
31. Townsend DJ, Lipp EB, Chun K, et al. Thumb duplication, 66 years experience: a review of surgical complications. J Hand Surg [Am] 1994; 19(6):973–6.
32. Manske PR. Treatment of duplicated thumb using a ligamentous/periosteal flap. J Hand Surg [Am] 1989;14(4):728–33.

33. Naasan A, Page RE. Duplication of the thumb; a 20-year retrospective review. J Hand Surg [Br] 1994; 19(3):355–60.

34. Bilhaut M. Guerison d'un pouce bifide par un nouveau procede operatoire. Conges Francais de Chirurgie 1889;4:576–80 [translated into English by Tonkin HE, Tonkin MA. Hand surgery, 1977;2:75–7].

35. Hartramph CR, Vasconez LO, Mathes S. Construction of one good thumb from both parts of a congenitally bifid thumb. Plast Reconstr Surg 1974;54(2): 148–52.

36. Tada K, Yonenobu K, Tsuyuguchi Y, et al. Duplication of the thumb: a retrospective review of two hundred and thirty seven cases. J Bone Joint Surg Am 1983; 65(5):584–98.

37. Dobyns JH, Lipscomb PR, Cooney WP. Management of thumb duplication. Clin Orthop Relat Res 1985;195:26–44.

38. Evans D. Polydactyly of the thumb. J Hand Surg [Br] 1993;18(1):3–4.

39. Tonkin MA, Bulstrode NW. The Bilhaut-Cloquet procedure for Wassel types III, IV and VII thumb duplication. J Hand Surg Eur Vol 2007;32(6):684–93.

40. Watson BT, Hennrikus WL. Postaxial type-B polydactyly. J Bone Joint Surg Am 1997;79(1):65–8.

41. Mohan J. Postaxial polydactyly in three Indian families. J Med Genet 1969;6(2):196–200.

42. Cantu JM, del Castillo V, Cortes R, et al. Autosomal recessive postaxial polydactyly: report of a family. Birth Defects Orig Artic Ser 1974;10(5):19–22.

43. Mollica F, Volti SL, Sorge G. Autosomal recessive postaxial polydactyly type A in a Sicilian family. J Med Genet 1978;15(3):212–6.

44. Merlob P, Grunebaum M, Reisner SH. A newborn infant with craniofacial dysmorphism and polysyndactyly (Greig's syndrome). Acta Paediatr Scand 1981;70(2):275–7.

45. Radhakrishna U, Blouin JL, Mehenni H, et al. Mapping one form of autosomal dominant postaxial polydactyly type A to chromosome 7p15-q11.23 by linkage analysis. Am J Hum Genet 1997;60(3): 597–604.

46. Akarsu AN, Stoilov I, Yilmaz E, et al. Genomic structure of HOXD13 gene: a nine polyalanine duplication causes synpolydactyly in two unrelated families. Hum Mol Genet 1996;5(7):945–52.

47. Zhao H, Tian Y, Breedveld G, et al. Postaxial polydactyly type A/B (PAP-A/B) is linked to chromosome 19p13.1–13.2 in a Chinese kindred. Eur J Hum Genet 2002;10(3):162–6.

48. Stelling F. The upper extremity. In: Fergusun AB, editor. Orthopaedic surgery in infancy and childhood. Baltimore (MD): Williams & Wilkins; 1963. p. 304–8.

49. Turek SL. Orthopaedic principles and their application. Philidelphia: J.B. Lippincott; 1967.

50. Temtamy SA, McKusick VA. The genetics of hand malformations. New York: Liss; 1978. p. 364.

51. Rayan GM, Frey B. Ulnar polydactyly. Plast Reconstr Surg 2001;107(6):1449–54.

52. Graham TJ, Ress AM. Finger polydactyly. Hand Clin 1998;14(1):49–64.

53. Tada K, Kurisaki E, Yonenobu K, et al. Central polydactyly-a review of 12 cases and their surgical treatment. J Hand Surg [Am] 1982;7(5):460–5.

54. Wood VE. Treatment of central polydactyly. Clin Orthop 1971;74:196–205.

55. Yang SS, Jackson L, Green DW, et al. A rare variant of mirror hand: a case report. J Hand Surg [Am] 1996;21(6):1048–51.

56. Al-Qattan MM, Al-Thunayan A, De Cordier M, et al. Classification of the mirror hand-multiple hand spectrum. J Hand Surg [Br] 1998;23B(4):534–6.

57. Saunders JW, Gasseling MT. Ectodermal-mesenchymal interactions in the origin of limb symmetry. In: Fleischmajer R, Billington RE, editors. Epithelial-mesenchymal interactions. Baltimore (MD): Williams & Wilkins; 1968. p. 78–97.

58. Tsuyuguchi Y, Tada K, Yonenobu K. Mirror hand anomaly: reconstruction of the thumb, wrist, forearm, and elbow. Plast Reconstr Surg 1982;70:384–7.

59. Pintilie D, Hatmanu D, Olaru I, et al. Double ulna with symmetrical polydactyly. J Bone Joint Surg Br 1964; 46:89–93.

Overgrowth Conditions: A Diagnostic and Therapeutic Conundrum

Matthew J. Carty, MD[a], Amir Taghinia, MD[b,c],
Joseph Upton, MD[b,d],*

KEYWORDS

- Overgrowth • Macrodactyly
- Lipomatous overgrowth
- Nerve territory oriented macrodactyly
- Lipomatosis • Gigantism
- Vascular malformations
- Proteus syndrome • Lipomatosis
- Parkes Weber syndrome
- Klippel-Trénaunay syndrome
- CLOVE syndrome

As a specific category, overgrowth problems in the hand and upper extremity occupy a very small proportion of congenital hand problems; but, when present, will challenge the most experienced hand surgeons. These constitute a wide spectrum of clinical phenotypes that contains very few common characteristics. Common to all of these hands is an overgrowth or a failure of differentiation of one or more cell types. Both skeletal and soft tissue elements may be involved in the growth process and, as the authors have learned, their maturation or senescence over time may not be normal. The mechanisms of overgrowth are not well understood.[1] As larger series of specific entities are accumulated, the natural history of many of these conditions will become clearer.

The purposes of this article are to (1) delineate characteristics of the specific clinical overgrowth conditions, (2) describe the growth patterns and clinical problems of each specific category of macrodactyly, and (3) outline the accepted principles of treatment.

CLASSIFICATION

In the past there has been no good classification system for hand overgrowth conditions; confusion has prevailed. Historically, many of these conditions were called hamartomas (Greek, *hamartia*, to sin), specific to malformed tissue that grew locally. The generic term macrodactyly (Greek, *macro*, large; *daktylos*, digit) has been used to describe situations in which there are enlarged digits. However, there exists a wide spectrum of overlapping conditions in which the entire limb and other parts of the body may also exhibit overgrowth. To add to this confusion, other common terms such as megalodactyly, gigantism, macrodystrophy lipomatosa, macrodactylia fibrolipomatosis, dactylomegaly, and gargantuan have appeared interchangeably in the literature.

Within hand surgery, a number of classification systems have been proposed but are changed as knowledge accumulates.[2–4] More recently, geneticists and interested pediatricians have

[a] Hand and Microsurgery, Beth Israel Deaconess Medical Center, Harvard Medical School, 31A Iroquois Street, Boston, MA 02120, USA
[b] Department of Surgery, Children's Hospital Boston, 300 Longwood Avenue, Hunnewell 1, Boston, MA 02115, USA
[c] Department of Surgery, Beth Israel Deaconess Medical Center, Harvard Medical School, Boston, MA, USA
[d] Shriners Hospital Boston, Harvard Medical School, Boston, MA, USA
* Corresponding author. 830 Boylston Street, Suite 212, Chestnut Hill, MA 02467.
E-mail address: jupton3@gmail.com (J. Upton).

Hand Clin 25 (2009) 229–245
doi:10.1016/j.hcl.2008.12.006
0749-0712/08/$ – see front matter © 2009 Elsevier Inc. All rights reserved.

organized what is known about the wide variety of overgrowth syndromes in a published book.[5] Working within this context, hand surgeons will encounter a number of conditions that may be characterized by overgrowth-related problems of the hand (**Table 1**). All but the rare and unusual forms of macrodactyly will fall into one of these nosologic categories. The present philosophy is to keep classification flexible and primarily based on clinical features until further progress in molecular genetics research has clarified understanding of these unusual problems.

CLINICAL PHENOTYPES AND THEIR NATURAL HISTORY
Nerve Territory-Oriented Macrodactyly and Lipomatous Macrodactyly

The majority of overgrowth problems seen by the hand surgeon falls into this group. The condition is unilateral 90% of the time. Males outnumber females by a 3:2 ratio and there is no familial inheritance. The affected thumb or digit is commonly asymmetrical, as the lipomatous overgrowth may follow either a median or ulnar nerve distribution within the hand—hence, the acronym NTOM (nerve territory-oriented macrodactyly).[6] Multiple digital involvement is much more common than overgrowth limited to an isolated digit or thumb. The affected digits or thumb will characteristically deviate away from one another and the palm is usually involved along the involved rays of the hand. There may be associated overgrowth and excessive fat accumulation within the arm and forearm and, commonly, large fat deposits will be present within the axilla with extension onto the chest wall. This fat distribution within the arm or forearm is either medial or lateral but is rarely completely circumferential. The skeletal changes show accelerated bone growth in length, width, and circumference at all levels. Epiphyses remain open through skeletal maturity but demonstrate moderate to severe asymmetry and greatly accelerated growth. Premature osteoarthritis develops within the affected portion of the limb. There are no abnormal skeletal lesions, osteochondromas, enchondromas, bone cysts, or assorted vascular malformations.

Two types of growth patterns are classically described: static and progressive; the distinction is made on clinical grounds.[7,8] The static type of enlargement is present at birth and the affected parts grow proportionally with the child. Surgical reduction and epiphysiodesis are usually performed later in childhood and the functional outcome is predictable. In the progressive type, overgrowth is usually present at birth and may be hard to distinguish from the static form. However, a slow, unrestricted, disproportionate thumb, digit, hand, or, occasionally, forearm or arm growth becomes obvious by age 2 to 3 years. Aggressive soft tissue and skeletal reduction is needed much earlier in life. Arthritic changes occur by the third decade of life. In a small number of patients, a third unrestricted type growth pattern is seen in which the affected parts are so large that early amputations are usually performed. Attempts at early, aggressive surgical reductions usually fail.

The tendons, intrinsic muscles, joints, and periarticular structures and skeletal parts are enlarged, but otherwise look normal. This is in contrast with other conditions such as Proteus syndrome, Maffucci syndrome, and vascular malformations. Lipomatous deposition surrounds all of these structures and may or may not involve segments of the peripheral nerves. The affected nerves within the palm are characteristically grossly enlarged; and compression neuropathies are common—particularly within the carpal canal, cubital tunnel, and radial tunnel. The fat within the forearm, elbow, and arm is primarily confined to the subcutaneous tissue planes, but may extend along fascial planes and between muscle groups. There is no infiltration of individual muscles or muscle groups; when this occurs, a different clinical condition is probably present. Despite the enlargement, muscle and joint function can be remarkably good. The size and bulk of the soft tissue enlargement are the greatest detriment to function in these hands and limbs. Sensation of the affected parts is normal early in life, but two-point discrimination and light touch inevitably become impaired because of unrecognized compression neuropathies, direct lipomatous infiltration of sensory nerves, thickened glabrous skin in palmar surfaces, or previous surgery including neurolysis or neurectomy. Incisions within the glabrous skin surfaces often become very hypertrophic.

Neurofibromatosis

Neurofibromatosis (NF) is not a common cause of macrodactyly, despite what has been reported in past hand literature. Fat proliferation is not predominant in this condition, in which unorganized overgrowth of the epineurium, perineurium, and endoneurium is seen. Although a generalized hyperplasia of a digit or thumb can occur, the enlargement seen represents soft tissue plexiform neurofibromas, schwannomas, and other types of nerve sheath tumors. The skin and subcutaneous tissue planes are primarily involved. Skeletal atrophy from disuse may be encountered in grossly enlarged limbs and hands. Malignant degeneration into fibrosarcomas can occur in extreme cases.[2]

Proteus Syndrome

In 1973, Widemann[9] described a syndrome with a bizarre collection of soft tissue and skeletal malformations and variable phenotypes. The name Proteus was fashioned after the Greek god who was gifted with the power of prophecy and the ability to change his form and appearance at will to avoid capture. No two patients are exactly alike, but most will have significant overgrowth of the hands or feet. Specific criteria for the diagnosis have been developed.[10] Many patients with overgrowth problems are universally misclassified as Proteus, because specific criteria such as macrodactyly can be found in other overgrowth syndromes.

The cerebriform, hyperkeratotic connective tissue appearance of the glabrous skin on the palms and soles is pathognomonic for this condition. Of specific interest to the hand surgeon is the progressive, asymmetric, often haphazard overgrowth of the thumb and digits. As the child grows, untreated overgrowth and secondary problems become worse. Cartilaginous masses originate in the palmar plates and the metacarpal heads and condyles of the phalanges are overgrown and asymmetrical. Joint stiffness, angulation, and rotational deformities develop. Flexion contractures are the major detriment to function and the hypertrophy of the palms and soles results in maceration, chronic infection, and persistent drainage. Within the overgrowth region, the flexor and extensor tendons, digital nerves, arteries, and intrinsic muscles are larger than normal. There is no significant lipomatous infiltration or accumulation. The most definitive characteristic of overgrowth in this condition is an unrelenting progression of growth. Early aggressive corrective surgery of the affected region of the extremity is recommended if function is to be maintained.

Multiple other conditions with similar skeletal changes such as exostoses, enlarged metacarpal heads, cartilaginous masses, enchondromas, and osteochondral masses adjacent to epiphyseal plates have been given labels such as hereditary exostoses. The thumb and digital configuration and growth may be bizarre and unpredictable and is the result of overgrowth of the skeletal parts and not the soft tissues. Further definition of this condition must await molecular analysis because many of these hands may be closely related genetically.

Hemihypertrophy or Hemihyperplasia

This category of macrodactyly is rare, difficult to describe, and not properly categorized within the hand literature. Geneticists have assigned many subsets to this condition.[11] Many prefer the term hemihyperplasia because this condition refers primarily to an increase in cell number, not cell size. Affected individuals usually present soon after birth with enlargement of one extremity. The overgrowth may involve a segmental region such as the face or the hand, or may affect the entire hemithorax and body. It is not localized to a single digit or thumb. The entire hand and palm may be less massive than other forms of overgrowth or gigantism. Common to all is skeletal overgrowth, metacarpal splaying, ulnar drift, and excessive digital length. Two clinical postures are generally noted. In the most common, the wrist is dorsiflexed, the digits are ulnar-deviated, and the thumb is flexed and adducted. A dynamic imbalance is created by increased tension from the extrinsic extensors and the intrinsic muscles, including the adductor pollicis muscle. The second posture is one of wrist flexion and ulnar deviation coupled with digital extension and thumb adduction. Exploration of both these enlarged forearms and hands has demonstrated abnormal, extra extrinsic muscle groups both on the flexor and extensor sides of the forearm, and a multitude of anomalous, atavistic intrinsic muscles within the hand. These muscle–tendon units do not have normal excursion and with growth cause progressive contractures, including the forearm flexors and extensors. When recognized early, these imbalances can be alleviated. When these patients present later in childhood or adolescence, skeletal alteration is the most effective way to correct the hand or wrist posture and improve functional outcomes.

Maffucci Syndrome and Ollier Disease

These conditions are characterized by multiple enchondromas with skeletal distortion together with vascular malformations, predominantly vascular malformations (VMs). These aberrations are most common in the hands and feet, but may involve any bone preformed from cartilage. The limb and hand deformities vary from moderate to marked and are always asymmetrical. These masses are to be distinguished from osteochondromas or exostoses and other cartilaginous growths commonly seen in Proteus syndrome. The designation Ollier disease is used when there are multiple enchondromas involving multiple bones. Early surgical excision of the VMs and enchondromas is effective and relatively easy, as these

Table 1

Comparison of overgrowth syndromes

	Klippel-Trénaunay Syndrome	Parkes Weber Syndrome	Lipomatous Overgrowth	CLOVE Syndrome	Hemihypertrophy	Proteus Syndrome	Maffucci syndrome
Capillary stain	Present, deep purple	Present, pink, often diffuse	Rare	Present, pink, diffuse, truncal	Uncommon	Present, pink, often diffuse	Absent (rarely reported)
Progressive overgrowth	Present	Present	Present, symmetric	Present, often extensive	Either overgrowth or undergrowth	Absent at birth, haphazard, unrelenting, disproportional	Secondary to enchondroma growth, moderate to massive
Hemodynamics	Slow-flow	Fast-flow	Slow-flow	Slow-flow	Slow-flow	Slow-flow	Slow-flow
Vascular anomalies	VM, LVM	AVM, AVF	Absent	VM, LVM, LM	Absent	VM, LM, CM	VM within bone, hands common
Associated anomalies	Common: GI, GU, genitalia	Rare, Cobb syndrome	Absent	No visceral	Skin, CNS, heart, GU, dental, others	Cerebriform soles/palms, linear nevi, dysregulated fat, lung cysts, facial neoplasms	None
Limb enlargement	Moderate, disproportionate digits and toes common	Arm, leg length discrepancy	Moderate, nerve territory-oriented	Moderate	Macrodactyly, syndactyly, polydactyly, club feet	Major, asymmetrical	Disproportionate
Limb affected	Upper 5%, lower 95%	Upper 23%, lower 77%	Equal	Equal	Arms, hands equally	Arms/legs, hands/feet equal	All
Skeletal changes	Unusual, can occur with large lesions	Common, direct involvement and demineralization	Common, symmetric	Marked scoliosis, lower limb	Hip dysplasia, scoliosis, increased bone age	Skull hyperostosis, vertebral megaspondylodysplasia	Gross distortion, asymmetry, limb length discrepancy, scoliosis, short stature, fractures
Macrodactyly	Diffuse enlargement	Minimal to moderate	Moderate to gigantic	Diffuse or longer with flexion contractures	Digits longer with flexion or extension contractures	Asymmetrical, moderate to gigantic	Digits longer with asymmetric masses, increased size due to tumors
Dysregulated fat	Present within malformation	Present	Common, entire limb and axilla	Present	Multiple lipomas	Lipomas, regional fat absence	Present occasionally
Nerve involvement	Absent	Absent	Intermittent	Intermittent	Absent, compression neuropathies with contractures	Absent	Absent

Muscle anomalies	None	Absent	Common, atavistic intrinsic and extrinsic muscles	Absent	Absent	Displaced by malformation	Displaced by VM, LVM
Associated neoplasms	Chondrosarcoma (17.5%–30%), many others les frequently (ovarian, CNS)	Ovarian, parotid	Renal, adrenal and CNS	Absent	Absent	Absent	Absent
Coagulopathy	None	Normal	Normal	Normal	Normal	Normal	Present
Cardiac failure	No	No	No	No	No	Yes	No
Clinical prognosis	Good with local therapy; Ollier disease patients demonstrate increased problems	Progressive growth of affected regions	Progressive flexion, extension and intrinsic contractures	Progressive deterioration with extensive limb involvement	Good, related to size and weight of limb	Often progressive deterioration, steal phenomenon. Prognosis is worse with CHF or amputation	Stable
Risks	Pathologic fractures	Neoplasms, PE, depression	Neoplasms (pheochromocytoma, Wilm's tumor, hepatoblastoma)	Scoliosis, pulmonary compromise	Secondary arthritis	Infection, CHF, gangrene	DVT risk increased post op
Genetics	Unknown	Unknown	Unknown	Unknown	Unknown	Unknown	Unknown

Abbreviations: AVM, arteriovenous malformation; CHF, congestive heart failure; CM, capillary malformation; CNS, central nervous system; DVT, deep vein thrombosis; GI, gastrointestinal; GU, genitourinary; LM, lymphatic malformation; LVM, lymphaticovenous malformation; PE, pulmonary embolism; VM, vascular malformations.

lesions shell out of their skeletal beds. Sclerotherapy is less effective because of the small size of these vascular channels.

Parkes Weber Syndrome

This form of macrodactyly, Parkes Weber (PW) syndrome, is easy to recognize because it is the only entity that involves a fast-flow vascular malformation. These hands are normal at birth and children usually present later in childhood with enlargement and minimal symptoms. Early symptoms of increased warmth and hyperhidrosis coupled with thrills and bruits should make the clinician suspicious. A capillary malformation (CM) is commonly present, in which case the designation capillary arteriovenous malformation is preferred over the eponym. The skeletal overgrowth seen is symmetric along the involved portion of the hand and is not as progressive and extensive as other forms described in this article. As these malformations progress and grow into more advanced clinical stages, one will see lytic lesions characteristic of direct skeletal invasion. Skeletal atrophy, demineralization, large lytic lesions, and pathologic fractures are seen with disuse with larger malformations. Early treatment emphasizes embolotherapy, and surgical debulking of these lesions within the hand is usually combined with preoperative embolization. The prognosis of these advanced lesions is very poor, as these lesions progress from one clinical stage to the next. The rate of progression is not predictable. The major risks are related to proximal shunting within the hand causing a distal steal phenomenon affecting the thumb or digits. Congestive heart failure can be the result of dynamic overload of the cardiopulmonary system by massive shunting within the extremity. Consumptive coagulopathies are not common.

Klippel-Trénaunay Syndrome

The limb or hand overgrowth in this condition is related to a slow-flow vascular malformation that may contain capillary, venous, lymphatic, or mixed venous-lymphatic channels. We prefer the designation of capillary-lymphaticovenous malformation (CLVM). All forms of macrodactyly within the upper limb have been misdiagnosed as Klippel-Trénaunay (KT) syndrome, which does have specific criteria. The increased size of the hand or extremity is secondary to skeletal elongation, and the hyperplasia of adipose tissue and vascular malformation. These are usually extensive lesions involving portions of the entire upper limb and are seen much more frequently in the lower extremity. The hands, forearms, and upper arms may be very large. Longitudinal growth of the limb may be decreased owing to epiphyseal involvement, but the size and bulk of the soft tissue can be increased to major proportions. Joint stiffness and contractures, compression neuropathies, and chronic pain become worse with growth. Skeletal atrophy is often seen in hands and arms. Conservative treatment and sclerotherapy are the initial treatments. Surgery is localized to specific problems, and symptomatic regions of the upper extremity and must be individualized. However, judicious soft tissue debulking, neurolysis, skeletal correction, growth-plate arrest, and other procedures can effectively improve the upper limb function in these children. The decision to operate is difficult and the technical expertise involved is quite challenging.

It is curious to note that both upper extremities may be involved and the malformation on the opposite side may be completely different. These limbs may not predominantly contain vascular malformations and may demonstrate enlarged muscle groups and hands similar to those described in the hemihypertrophy section. Digits are long and flexed at the metacarpophalangeal (MP) joints and there may be some ulnar drift or a "windblown" posture. The rays of these hands are splayed apart.

New Phenotype

Within the past year, a separate group of overgrowth patients previously designated as suffering from either Proteus or KT syndrome has been described. This new phenotype, known as CLOVE syndrome, includes capillary (C) malformations, lipomatous overgrowth (LO) of the trunk or extremities, vascular malformations (VM), epidermal (E) nevi, and skeletal distortions.[12] More recently, central nervous system (CNS) malformations and seizure have been added to this clinical entity.[13] This may involve a small portion of a hand or foot, but more commonly includes the entire limb. The adipose deposits are substantial and peripheral nerves may or may not be infiltrated. The overgrowth of the tubular bones in the extremities is progressive but not as haphazard as that seen in the Proteus syndrome or gigantic types of lipomatous macrodactyly. Those limbs with vascular malformations are quite similar to KT syndrome patients and, indeed, may be genetically related. Treatment is similar to KT syndrome patients. With arm and truncal involvement, scoliosis may be present and without skeletal stabilization becomes more severe with growth. The feet may be characteristically oversized with splayed toes and massive soft tissue deformation involving the dorsal or plantar surfaces.

PRINCIPLES OF MANAGEMENT

The diversity of phenotypes associated with overgrowth of the hand renders the notion of approaching the treatment of these patients through algorithms or other formulaic strategies impossible. Surgical management of individuals suffering from hand overgrowth demands ingenuity and technical virtuosity from the reconstructive hand surgeon because no two patients are ever alike, the problems posed are not normal, and effective therapy generally requires aggressive—rather than piecemeal—interventions.

Treatment decisions for these patients therefore require thoughtful consideration of both the reasons for intervention and the objectives of therapy. The primary indications for intervening in upper limb overgrowth scenarios are intuitive—namely, when such conditions are associated with gross impairment in function (namely prehension and grip) or appearance. The goals of therapy parallel these indications and include: (1) enabling optimal hand function through the establishment or preservation of meaningful grip, pinch, and precise prehension; and (2) providing an aesthetic limb that approximates the appearance of a typical adult hand.

Many techniques have been promoted for the surgical management of hand overgrowth. While applauding the efforts of our predecessors and contemporaries alike who have contributed to this war chest of operative procedures (some with dire outcomes), the authors instead advocate an approach to therapy based on surgical principles developed over 30 years of treating patients who suffer from overgrowth disorders. Surgical principles gain popularity with time but must be continually reassessed and refined, while surgical techniques change more rapidly, are affected by advancing technology, and require constant reevaluation. Adherence to the following principles in the preoperative planning phases, as well as in the intraoperative execution, cannot be overemphasized.

Planning

Careful preoperative planning should include consideration of the age of the patient, clinical phenotype, associated comorbidities, severity and extent of deformity, maturation stage of digit, digital range of motion, and the desires and expectations of both the patient and his or her family. All studies should be reviewed preoperatively; serial radiographic studies of growing children are often invaluable in demonstrating the true extent of involvement of the extremity. MRI scans have become the gold standard for evaluation of vascular malformations in both the diagnostic- and treatment-planning processes. A thorough explanation of all potential complications must be given to the patient and parents, including diminished sensation, stiffness, and arthritis.

Timing

When indicated, operative intervention should be planned as early as possible. Skeletal growth arrest should ideally be timed to coincide with the point at which the involved digit is the same size as that of the equivalent digit on the same-sex parent; however, debulking and remodeling procedures may be performed at any time. A disproportionately large digit should not be allowed to go untreated through school ages, as psychological issues are significant concerns in the growing child and young adolescent (**Fig. 1**).

Amputation

If the decision for digital salvage is made, both skeletal and soft tissue debulking should be pursued aggressively to optimize both function and appearance. When the anticipated outcome from reconstruction is likely to be unacceptable, amputation should be considered early and discussed at length due to the difficulty and variable outcomes of reduction procedures.

Incisions

The placement of incisions is important—particularly in children. A high midaxial incision in the digit is preferred, as it can be used many times and is hidden. With growth, volar scars in or near the palm can lead to contracture. If a palmar approach is chosen, a zigzag incision is preferred. Palmar incisions in vascular malformations, Proteus syndrome patients, and lipomatous overgrowth have a predilection to atrophy.

Tourniquet Usage

All dissection should be performed with the aid of a pneumatic tourniquet to optimize visualization and identification of key structures in a bloodless field.

Magnification

The use of magnification, either loupe or microscope, makes a tremendous difference in the identification and preservation of normal neurovascular structures. Small vessels such as vincular pedicles to the flexor tendons, the palmar arches, and nutrient vessels to the carpal bones should be saved if uninvolved. Meticulous technique and compulsive hemostasis will obviate

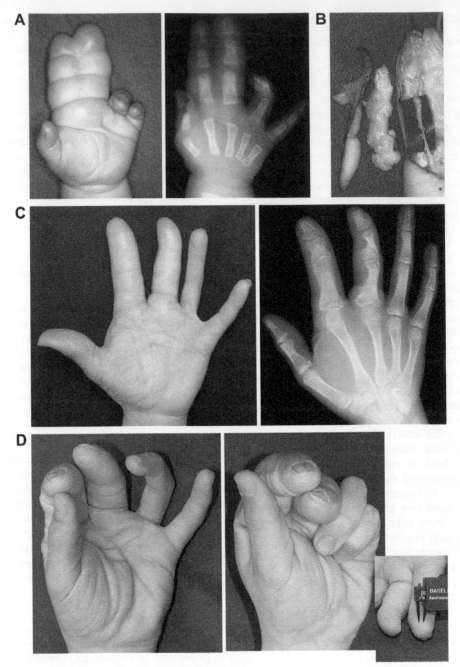

Fig. 1. Lipomatous overgrowth. (*A*) The clinical appearance and radiograph of a 3-month-old child with massive enlargement of the index and long digits joined by a simple complete syndactyly. (*B*) Early aggressive separation was performed in stages. The debulking on the radial side of the index digits included skin and soft tissue removal and a microvascular dissection of the neurovascular bundle. Note the lack of lipomatous involvement of the digital nerve. A longitudinal reduction of the phalanges with reconstruction of a collateral ligament was also performed. (*C*) Epiphysiodeses were performed when the phalanges were close to adult length and compensation was made for extra metacarpal length. Note the increased width and circumference of these phalanges. The patient is 19 years of age. (*D*) At 21 years of age the same patient has retained digits with some limitation of motion at the proximal interphalangeal joints and very little motion at the distal interphalangeal joint level. Moving two-point discrimination is 8.0 mm—higher than normal, but less than protective levels. Despite aggressive debulking, the overall size of these digits is larger than normal. However, the patient and family are very pleased with this outcome.

the difficulties inherent to dissecting in a blood-stained field.

Blood Supply

To avoid vascular compromise, only half of a digit should be dissected at a time. If possible, at least one or two large dorsal veins per finger should be preserved. When a critical arterial segment to a digit is resected, this segment should be reconstructed with a vein graft so that at least one digital artery is preserved per digit.

Motion

Every effort should be made to preserve metacarpophalangeal joint motion.

Sensibility

Radical debulking of the pulp on the ulnar side of the thumb and radial side of the index finger is not advised owing to the risk of compromising pinch sensibility.

Thorough Surgery

Debulking procedures extending into the palm or any other region should be thorough to avoid the need for surgical re-entry into a densely scarred bed.

Tension

Skin flaps should not be inset under tension, and nonviable skin should be replaced with skin grafts or a flap. Tissue with questionable viability can be observed and resected later, if necessary.

Drains

Drains should be used liberally, and delayed primary closure of the surgical wound should be considered. Persistent postoperative bleeding is usually best treated with direct pressure, elevation, and immobilization, rather than with re-exploration. Tissue sealant products are especially useful with vascular malformations.

Follow-up

Regardless of the particular type of overgrowth disorder, follow-up evaluation should be performed compulsively at yearly intervals.

THERAPEUTIC TECHNIQUES

There is no useful nonsurgical treatment for overgrowth disorders of the upper extremity. Although compression bandaging may be a helpful adjunct to surgical intervention in cases of overgrowth related to vascular malformations (eg, PW, KT, or CLOVE syndrome) or as a means for limiting digital swelling, it is not a curative, definitive therapy. Minimally invasive approaches to limit skeletal overgrowth through embolization therapy may become a reality as interventional radiology techniques continue to advance. At present, however, such modalities remain limited to large bones only.[14]

Over the past century, a myriad of surgical procedures has been described to remedy the functional and aesthetic concerns related to hand overgrowth disorders. It is beyond the scope of this article to survey all of the techniques noted in the literature. Instead, the authors will provide a broad overview of available options based on whether the principle reconstructive effort is designed to effect salvage through soft tissue or skeletal reduction, amputation, or replacement of the involved digit.

Digital Salvage

Surgical preservation of an overgrown digit may be achieved by growth arrest, skeletal or soft tissue reduction, or a combination. In general, growth arrest procedures limited to soft tissue manipulation alone have proven ineffective. Indeed, follow up studies detailing the long-term outcomes of techniques including digital artery ligation and digital nerve stripping or resection have demonstrated little to no effect on growth cessation in digital overgrowth conditions.[15,16]

Growth arrest through epiphysiodesis is a well-demonstrated and reliable method of terminating longitudinal digital skeletal overgrowth. Although a variety of techniques for achieving epiphysiodesis by way of drilling or physeal stapling have been described, our preferred method is to perform multilevel epiphyseal plate resections using an osteotome or dental bur to provide complete growth ablation throughout the affected phalanx or metacarpal. Many patients with Proteus syndrome, CLOVE syndrome, and lipomatous overgrowth require epiphysiodesis or forearm ostectomy to control wrist deviation and malalignment. Regardless of the technique performed, skeletal growth arrest should be timed to occur at the point at which the involved digit has reached a length equivalent to that of the analogous digit in the patient's same-sex adult parent. Epiphysiodesis accomplishes growth arrest in the longitudinal direction only; correction of disproportionate digital width and circumference must be addressed through other techniques, as described below.

Procedures designed to achieve phalangeal reduction comprise a second category of interventions available for digital salvage. In cases in which reconstructive needs are limited to debulking of soft tissues only, we favor a high midlateral approach over a palmar zigzag incision because of the higher incidence of scar hypertrophy and contracture in this patient population. Debulking procedures may safely involve the entire length of a digit; however, such procedures should be limited to one side of a digit at a time to limit the potential for vascular compromise, with a latency period of at least three to six months before operating on the opposite side. We preserve the digital arteries, vincular branches and entire palmar arch through meticulous microsurgical dissection. While epiphysiodesis is a time-sensitive procedure, soft tissue debulking may be performed at any time. Following microsurgical neuroplasty and pulp reduction, the remaining palmar skin will be reinnervated by the axonal sprouting from the remaining digital nerve.

The authors advocate early and aggressive staged soft tissue debulking to achieve a digit whose appearance and function is as normal as possible before a patient reaches school age. Requiring a young child to advance through the childhood years with a grotesquely enlarged limb or digit should be avoided.

Phalangeal reduction efforts requiring both skeletal *and* soft tissue remodeling may be based upon a number of well-described eponymous procedures.[7,17–23] No single procedure should be applied uniformly, and the selection of the appropriate technique for correction of a given digit must be tailored to the specific reconstructive problems posed. Important considerations include the involved digit, the axis of the digit requiring reduction, the necessity for growth arrest and at what levels, the preservation of motion and at what level, and the requirement for nail recontouring and pulp reduction (**Fig. 2**, **Table 2**). All techniques resulting in longitudinal reduction require tendon rebalancing to maximize function and many soft tissue and nail procedures must be completed in stages.

Digital Amputation

In severe cases of digital overgrowth, the most experienced hand surgeon has little hope of attaining a reasonable functional and aesthetic result through digital salvage. However, these are not impossible problems and reconstruction should be considered for minimal and moderate deformities. The potential self esteem issues of the child should be carefully monitored during the early formative years. When appropriate, options for digital amputation should be considered early and discussed at length with the parents. The use of pre- and postoperative hand molds is especially helpful in these situations.[24] When amputation is warranted, neither the hand surgeon nor the patient or family should perceive this situation as a therapeutic failure, as the end result of such a measure may result in a better functional, aesthetic, and psychosocial outcome than what is achievable through other treatment modalities.

When severe overgrowth is limited to the distal digit, terminalization of the phalanx may be performed using resection osteotomy to achieve appropriate length followed by tailoring of the distal soft tissue envelope. In extreme cases of overgrowth, this requires concomitant sacrifice of the nail plate and nail bed and recontouring of the tip pulp. When overgrowth involves the entire digit, either a complete ray resection or transmetacarpal amputation may be considered. Special attention should be paid to preserving the vascular and neurosensory integrity of the remaining digits in such cases, because the underlying anatomy is often displaced or distorted. In such circumstances, microvascular dissection techniques should be employed. Amputation should include resection of as much associated skin as possible, because this tissue is not normal and may demonstrate unpredictable healing behavior. When required, full thickness skin grafts should supplement closure efforts.

Digital Replacement

The continued evolution of microsurgical techniques has enabled the reconstruction of severely overgrown digits through the employment of free toe transfers. The primary indication for digital replacement is for reconstruction of a grotesquely overgrown thumb requiring amputation to the level of the metacarpal. In such cases, an excellent functional and aesthetic result is possible through microsurgical transfer of the great toe according to well-described techniques.[25] When possible, we advise toe transfer at the time of amputation. With the application of meticulous microsurgical technique and aggressive postoperative hand therapy, good range of motion and sensibility may be achieved, dramatically enhancing the function and appearance of an otherwise severely impaired hand. A hand containing a thumb plus one or two additional digits can provide a very functional and aesthetically acceptable reconstructive outcome (**Fig. 3**).

OUTCOMES

Very few, if any, of the illustrations in current textbooks adequately portray this deformity as it actually exists; and case reports and large series do

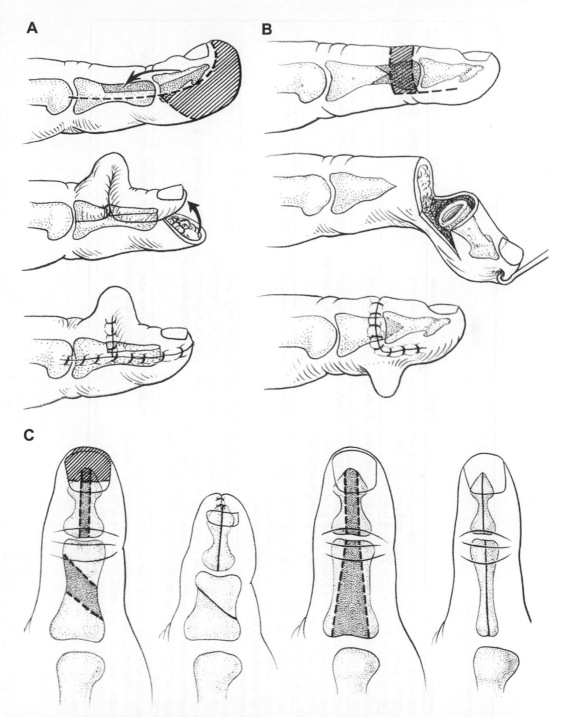

Fig. 2. Skeletal reduction. (*A*) One type of reduction of the massive fingertip involves aggressive pulp resection, isolation of the remaining nail complex including dorsal cortex of the distal phalanx as a dorsal pedicle, and transfer on top of the middle phalanx. (*B*) Another strategy involves bone resection, dorsal skin and tendon resection, and transfer as a palmar pedicle. The skin excess in both methods is removed secondarily. (*C*) For massive thumb overgrowth, skeletal reduction can be achieved with longitudinal, oblique, or central longitudinal excisions. Motion at the interphalangeal joint is invariably diminished or completely lost as these children grow and develop secondary osteoarthritis. (*From* Upton J. Failure of differentiation and overgrowth. In: Mathes SJ, Hentz VR, editors. Plastic Surgery. 2nd edition. Volume VIII: The hand and upper limb, Part 2. Philadelphia: WB Saunders; 2005. p. 301, 302, 305, 315; with permission.)

Table 2
Comparison of phalangeal reduction techniques

Treatment Eponym (Year Coined)	Description	Digit	Axis of Reduction	Growth Arrest	Motion Reduction
Barsky (1967)	Resection of distal part of middle phalanx, distal phalanx articular surface and growth plate, and conical distal phalangeal core to fit middle phalanx resection	Phalanx	Longitudinal only	Distal phalanx only	Sacrifices DIP joint motion
Tsuge (1967)	Resection of all phalangeal growth plates in conjunction with tipplasty	Phalanx	Longitudinal only	All levels	None
Hoshi (1973)	Resection osteotomy of proximal metacarpal, DIP joint resection osteotomy and fusion, distal phalangeal tip resection osteotomy, unilateral digital longitudinal soft tissue wedge resection	Phalanx	Longitudinal and modest transverse	Distal phalanx only	Sacrifices DIP joint motion
Millesi (1974)	Resection of distal phalanx distally and along central longitudinal strip combined with shortening of proximal phalanx by way of oblique resection osteotomy	Thumb	Longitudinal only	None	None
Fujita (1983)	Resection osteotomy of distal phalanx tip in conjunction with tip and unilateral digital soft tissue resection	Phalanx	Longitudinal and modest transverse	None	None
Ogino (1998)	Resection osteotomy of proximal phalanx, DIP joint resection osteotomy and fusion, distal phalanx tip resection osteotomy, tip and unilateral digital soft tissue resection	Phalanx	Longitudinal and modest transverse	Distal phalanx only	Sacrifices DIP joint motion
Bertelli (2001)	Resection osteotomy of DIP join with concomitant unilateral longitudinal resection osteotomies of distal, middle and distal proximal phalanges with tip and unilateral digital soft tissue resection	Phalanx	Longitudinal and substantial transverse	Distal phalanx only	Sacrifices DIP joint motion

Abbreviation: DIP, distal interphalangeal joint.

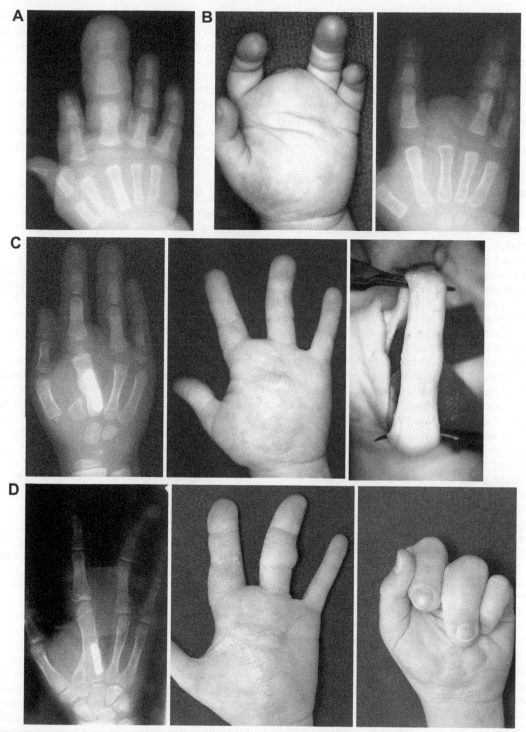

Fig. 3. Amputation. (*A*) Amputation of this massively enlarged long digit was performed within the first year of life. (*B*) When the child was referred at 2 years of age, massive lipomatous enlargement of the palm was prominent and there was a noticeable gap between the index and ring digits. The numbness in the median nerve distribution was secondary to compressive of a massively enlarged nerve. (*C*) At age 3 years, a transposition of the index to long was performed. Subsequent debulkings and epiphysiodeses of the adjacent index and ring digits and a complete debulking of the palm were completed. (*D*) At age 23 years, the patient has maintained excellent motion at the MP and PIP joint levels. Motion at the DIP level is significantly reduced.

not show long-term postoperative results, which are never normal. All described series are small, and most contain a long list of different conditions as outlined before. No treatment is entirely satisfactory. The authors' experience with a large number of these patients treated during the past 30 years is summarized by specific condition. At present, the literature does not contain any long term follow up or specific outcomes data for any of these conditions.

Nerve Territory-Oriented Macrodactyly and Lipomatous Macrodactyly

The nerve territory-oriented macrodactyly, with or without neural infiltration and lipomatous macrodactylies, have similar outcomes. When motion is deficient because of sheer bulk, it is not improved postoperatively. Those with localized digit or thumb involvement will retain excellent sensation and will retain satisfactory motion. Outcomes with those patients exhibiting the static growth pattern are predictably better than those demonstrating the progressive and unrestricted patterns. Length is controlled with appropriate epiphyseal obliteration, but the circumference is always greater than in uninvolved digits. The skeletal deviation will recur unless the entire growth plate of the involved phalanx or metacarpal is obliterated. Incisions in the glabrous skin of the digit are routinely more hypertrophied than high midaxial incisions. Amputation of grossly enlarged digits or thumb is a good option. Microvascular great-toe transfer is preferable to multistaged debulking of the thumb ray (**Fig. 4**).

As these growing children are observed, attention must be directed to additional palmar, forearm, or arm enlargement, which may progressively increase. There is a misconception that sensation is or can be normal in these patients. With the exception of those with minimal involvement, moving and static two-point discrimination is always impaired. After repeated debulking and nerve manipulation, protective sensation, at best, will result. If they are observed long enough through adolescence into adulthood, most of these patients will develop clinical and radiologic signs of a progressive osteoarthritis in the involved portions of the hand. The authors do not know if previous debulking or contouring can alter this process but are beginning to see early arthritis in toes transferred into these regions. Close observation of more than 100 patients following debulking is currently in progress.

Neurofibromatosis

Neurofibromatosis is present in a very small group of overgrowth patients. Minimal hand and forearm deformities should not affect existing hand function. Compression neuropathies at the wrist and elbow levels respond to appropriate decompression but are often overlooked in children who have adapted and learned to avoid cuts, abrasions, and infections. Extensive arm, forearm, and hand lesions can be debulked for functional reasons with predictable outcomes. Malignant degeneration is a concern in these extremities and has been seen in our practice five times during the last 30 years.

Proteus Syndrome

The hand deformities in those with Proteus syndrome and congenital hyperostosis are rare and have similar outcomes. The skeletal malformations and large cartilaginous masses that involve joint spaces are the cause of diminished motion and rotational or angulation deformities. Surgery along the digits or thumb invariably results in a loss of motion, which is proportional to the extent of the deformity. Incisions involving the glabrous skin become hypertrophic, and the cerebriform fibrous overgrowth must be removed and resurfaced if the involved digit, thumb, or hand is to be functional. Sensation is not normal in these hands because of the thickness of the outer skin layers. Unrelenting, progressive growth often makes the affected portions of the hand minimally functional. In many severely involved individuals, the upper limb manifestations are often understandably given a much lower priority for treatment than other life-threatening malformations.

Hemihypertrophy or Hemihyperplasia

Because there is such a wide variation of hand findings in those with hemihypertrophy, outcome studies do not exist. Most of these hands are amazingly functional despite the deformities caused by hypertrophic and atavistic muscle groups resulting in various flexion contractures of the forearm and hand and ulnar deviation of the digits. Every case must be carefully individualized. Surgical decisions are dictated by functional and aesthetic needs. In many patients, there has been no loss of function with removal of hypertrophied muscle groups in the hand and forearm. Ulnar deviation of digits is not always reversed by early or late release of tight intrinsic muscles. Wrist and digital flexion contractures secondary to tight extrinsic flexor tendons are improved only by complete tenotomies instead of tendon lengthening. These muscles are nonfunctional, have little passive excursion, and, with growth, contribute to progressively worsening functional status. Excessive ulnar deviation and widening of

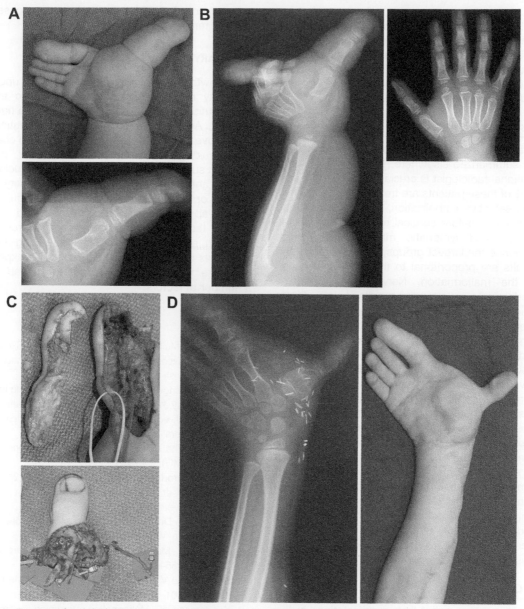

Fig. 4. Toe transfer. (*A*) This 15 month-old child was referred with massive enlargement of the radial side of the hand. The thumb and index digit were heavy, stiff and nonfunctional. (*B*) The soft tissue enlargement continues up the entire radial (lateral) side of the forearm, elbow, and arm into the axilla. Note the skeletal overgrowth in all three dimensions. The comparison to the unaffected opposite hand is dramatic. The family wished desperately to have these enlarged parts amputated. (*C*) A compromise was reached. The index digit was saved with aggressive soft tissue and skeletal resection at age 2 years, and the thumb was amputated and replaced with a modified great toe transfer. One year later, the entire palm was debulked and the median nerve decompressed. (*D*) The same limb is seen six years later before a closing wedge osteotomy of the radius. Soft tissue debulking has extended up to and including the axilla. The hand is very functional and the appearance is definitely improved. This child does not hide her abnormal hand. Note the early arthritic changes in the affected index digit age 9 years. Unaffected dorsal sensory branches of the radial nerve were used to innervate the toe transfer. The moving two-point discrimination on both sides of this thumb is 8.0 mm, and the patient perceives this as palmar pulp sensation.

the hand are best corrected with metacarpal osteotomies. Normal extrinsic and intrinsic muscles of the limb should be left untouched because diminution of excursion and weakness will invariably result from surgical manipulation. Progressive joint deformities will not be corrected with hand therapy and splinting alone.

Vascular Malformations

Outcomes of those with vascular malformations are summarized elsewhere. The role of the interventional radiologist is crucial because more than 80% of these patients are treated with sclerotherapy, selective embolization, or other specialized techniques before surgical resection. In general, venous and lymphatic malformations, which comprise the largest groups, are resectable, and results are proportional to the size and location of the malformation. Nerve-related problems predominate in untoward results. Large, diffuse lesions with or without lymphatic components seen in patients with the Klippel-Trénaunay syndrome (CLVM) are the most difficult to treat, and results are never normal. Localized or high-flow lesions, fortunately, are rare. Embolization followed by complete excision and revascularization, if necessary, is effective in the short run. If observed long enough (more than 20 years), most of these lesions recur in adjacent regions and become problematic. Lymphatic malformations respond well to surgery, and function is not as severely affected as with other malformations primarily because most of these lesions are confined to the skin and subcutaneous tissue planes.[24] Hypertrophic scars, continued swelling, and joint stiffness plague these patients. Small, localized lesions are easily removed without any loss of function.

CLOVE Syndrome

The hand and upper limb manifestations in this condition vary and outcomes are similar to those in the specific groups. However, the overgrowth patterns in this unique set of patients tend to be dramatic. A CLOVE syndrome child with a venous malfomation or lymphatic malfomation will have a large, diffuse lesion with impressive overgrowth that may involve two to three digits and extend into the forearm or even the axilla. When necessary, repositioning of the shoulder and elbow to achieve maximal hand and wrist function should be considered before any hand surgery. Outcomes in all categories are in the fair to good range. Despite the fact that these patients often struggle with issues related to limb overgrowth throughout their lives, they generally begin to adapt shortly following birth and, in many cases, achieve remarkable levels of function.

SUMMARY

Overgrowth conditions involving the upper extremity represent a complex diagnostic and therapeutic challenge for the reconstructive hand surgeon. Advances in genetics research continue to improve our capacity to both classify and characterize discrete overgrowth conditions, and assist in surgical planning through better elucidation of anticipated natural history. A variety of surgical options exist. Selection should be guided by the application of core principles and may include techniques dedicated to digital reconstruction, amputation, or replacement. Long-term outcomes based on 30 years of operative experience are fair to good, and are influenced by a number of factors.

REFERENCES

1. Boyd JB, Mulliken JB, Kaban LB, et al. Skeletal changes associated with vascular malformations. Plast Reconstr Surg 1984;74:789–97.
2. Upton J. Congenital anomalies of the hand and forearm. In: May JW Jr, Littler JW, editors. The Hand. In: McCarthy J, editor. Plastic surgery, 8. Philadelphia: WB Saunders; 1990.
3. Flatt AE. The care of congenital hand anomalies. St. Louis (MO): CV Mosby; 1977.
4. Dell P. Macrodactyly. Hand Clin 1985;1:511–24.
5. Cohen MM Jr. Overgrowth syndromes. New York: Oxford University Press; 2002.
6. Kelikian H. Deformities of the hand and forearm. Philadelphia: WB Saunders; 1974.
7. Barksy AJ. Macrodactyly. J Bone Joint Surg Am 1967;49:1255–66.
8. De Laurenzi V. Macrodattilia de medio. G Med Mil 1962;112:401–5 [in Italian].
9. Wiedemann HR. Malformation-retardation syndrome with bilateral absence of the 5th rays in both hand and feet, cleft palate, malformed ears and eyelids, radioulnar synostosis. Klin Padiatr 1973;185:181–6 [in German].
10. Biesecker L, Happle R, Mulliken JB, et al. Proteus syndrome: diagnostic criteria, differential diagnosis and patient evaluation. Am J Med Genet 1999;84:389–95.
11. Cohen MM Jr. Perspectives on overgrowth syndromes. Am J Med Genet 1998;79:234–7.
12. Sapp JC, Turner JT, van de Kamp JM, et al. Newly delineated syndrome of congenital lipomatous overgrowth, vascular malformations and epidermal nevi (CLOVE syndrome) in seven patients. Am J Med Genet 2007;143A:2944–58.

13. Gucev ZS, Tasic V, Jancevska A, et al. Congenital lipomatous overgrowth, vascular malformations, and epidermal nevi (CLOVE) syndrome: CNS malformations and seizures may be a component of this disorder. Am J Med Genet A 2008;146A(20): 2688–90.

14. Egerszegi EP. Congenital hand anomalies: overgrowth. In: Bentz ML, Bauer BS, Zuker RM, editors. Principles and practice of pediatric plastic surgery. St. Louis (MO): Quality Medical Publishing; 2008.

15. Flatt AE. Large fingers. In: Flatt AE, editor. The care of congenital hand anomalies. 2nd edition. St. Louis (MO): Quality Medical Publishing; 1994.

16. Tsuge K. Treatment of macrodactyly. J Hand Surg [Am] 1985;10:968–9.

17. Tsuge K. Treatment of macrodactyly. Plast Reconstr Surg 1967;39:590–9.

18. Hoshi E, Tajima T, Watanabe Y. Results of our treatment of macrodactyly. Keisei Geka 1973;24:1183–9.

19. Millesi H. Macrodactyly: as case study. In: Littler J, Carrner L, Smith J, editors. Symposium on reconstructive hand surgery. St. Louis (MO): CV Mosby; 1974.

20. Fujita S, Kodoma K, Watanabe H. Treatment of macrodactyly. Keisei Geka 1983;26:420–5.

21. Ogino T. Macrodactyly. In: Buck-Gramcko D, editor. Congenital malformations of the hand and forearm. Toronto: Churchill-Livingstone; 1998.

22. Bertelli JA, Pigozzi L, Pereima M. Hemidigital resection with collateral ligament transplantation in the treatment of macrodactyly: a case report. J Hand Surg [Am] 2001;26:623–7.

23. Tan O, Atik B, Dogan A, et al. Middle phalangectomy: a functional and aesthetic cure for macrodactyly. Scand J Plast Reconstr Surg Hand Surg 2006;40:362–5.

24. Upton J. Failure of differentiation and overgrowth. In: Mathes SJ, Hentz VR, editors. Plastic surgery. 2nd edition, VIII. The hand and upper limb, Part 2. Philadelphia: WB Saunders; 2005.

25. Upton J, Mutimer K. A modification of the great-toe transfer for thumb reconstruction. Plast Reconstr Surg 1988;82:535–8.

Undergrowth: Brachydactyly

Michael L. Nguyen, MD[a], Neil F. Jones, MD[b],*

KEYWORDS

- Brachydactyly • Distraction lengthening
- Toe-to-hand transfers • Congenital hand
- Undergrowth

At its simplest, brachydactyly is the Greek word for "short finger," but essentially it describes digital hypoplasia or aplasia. The index and small fingers are the most commonly affected digits, and the middle phalanx is the most commonly affected bone. It is frequently inherited in an autosomal dominant fashion and can be associated with numerous congenital syndromes, including Treacher Collins, Apert, Poland, Cornelia de Lange and Bloom syndromes.[1] Congenital constriction ring syndrome also produces brachydactyly, but this is discussed in another article elsewhere in this issue. Similarly, hypoplasia of the thumb also warrants its own separate article.

Presentation of brachydactyly is highly variable. Digits may be normal in proportion yet hypoplastic, or a digit can fail to form any of the phalanges and/or the metacarpal, or the digit may present as complete aplasia. The deformity may be associated with either a longitudinal deficiency, such as in radial and ulnar longitudinal deficiencies, or a transverse deficiency, such as congenital constriction ring syndrome and symbrachydactyly. Several terms have been used to describe the variable presentations, many of which are purely semantic and have no real benefit to the surgeon. Ectrodactyly is a general term that describes the complete absence of phalanges or a metacarpal. A shortened metacarpal is termed "brachymetacarpia" (**Fig. 1**), and a short phalanx is termed "brachyphalangia" (**Fig. 2**). Brachyphalangia may be further classified into which bone is shortened. A short proximal phalanx is termed "brachybasophalangia," a short middle phalanx is termed "brachymesophalangia," and a short distal phalanx is termed "brachytelephalangia."

CLASSIFICATION

Bell's classification of congenital hand anomalies in 1951 is the standard by which brachydactyly is organized.[1] Unfortunately, this classification system does not help surgeons to plan treatment, but it does help geneticists to assess inheritance risk patterns. Most hand surgeons use the classification system described by Swanson and adopted by the American Society for Surgery of the Hand and the International Federation of Societies for Surgery of the Hand.[2] Undergrowth is one of the seven separate categories in this classification system.

Symbrachydactyly has its own classification system described by Blauth and Gekeler,[3] which identifies four types:

> Peromelic: a transverse amputation at the level of the metacarpals
> Oligodactylic: the central portion of the hand is aplastic
> Short finger: the four fingers are shortened and not fully differentiated, although the thumb is relatively normal
> Monodactylic: a finger is aplastic but the thumb is relatively normal

Most patients with brachydactyly, especially cases that involve just one phalanx, do not require any surgical intervention; they are of interest to pediatricians and geneticists only. As the degree of brachydactyly in a single ray becomes more severe and

a Department of Orthopedic Surgery, University of California-Irvine Medical Center, 101 The City Drive South, Pavilion III, Room 210, Orange, CA 92868, USA
b Department of Orthopedic Surgery, Division of Plastic and Reconstructive Surgery, University of California-Irvine Medical Center, 101 The City Drive South, Pavilion III, Room 210, Orange, CA 92868, USA
* Corresponding author.
E-mail address: nfjones@uci.edu (N.F. Jones).

Hand Clin 25 (2009) 247–255
doi:10.1016/j.hcl.2009.02.003
0749-0712/09/$ – see front matter © 2009 Published by Elsevier Inc.

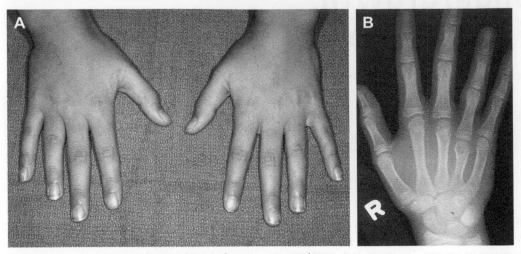

Fig. 1. (*A, B*) Brachymetacarpia of the right ring finger metacarpal.

results in severe hypoplasia or complete aplasia of a digit or if the brachydactyly involves multiple digits, however, hand function becomes compromised and the child should be considered for surgical reconstruction. Surgical treatment for brachydactyly may improve function and appearance, but function always takes precedence. Current surgical treatment options include web space deepening, osteotomy and immediate interposition bone grafting (**Fig. 3**), nonvascularized toe phalangeal bone grafting, distraction lengthening, and microsurgical toe-to-hand transfers. Historically, metacarpal or phalangeal transfer ("on-top plasty") was popular, but it has fallen out of favor because results have been less than optimal. The results of the conventional techniques of nonvascularized toe phalangeal bone grafting and distraction lengthening and the newer technique of microsurgical toe-to-hand transfers are discussed.

NONVASCULARIZED TOE PHALANGEAL BONE GRAFTS

Nonvascularized toe phalangeal bone grafts have been advocated for hypoplastic digits consisting essentially of "skin tubes" to provide length and stability. Results have varied, from the bone graft being completely resorbed to satisfactory epiphyseal growth without resorption. Unfortunately, various series have demonstrated the results to be inconsistent, although they have improved considerably since extraperiosteal harvesting of the toe phalanx has become standard.

The first nonvascularized toe phalangeal bone graft was reported by Noesske in 1919 and later by Entin in 1959,[4] but this surgical option did not receive much attention until Goldberg and Watson[5] recognized the importance of harvesting

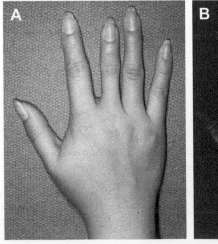
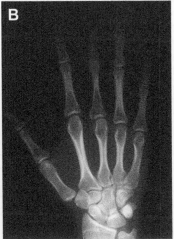

Fig. 2. (*A, B*) Brachyphalangia of the middle phalanx of the right middle finger.

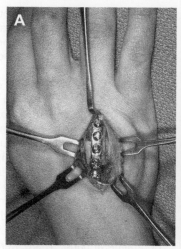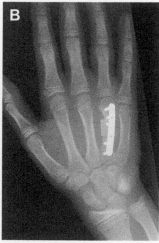

Fig. 3. (A, B) Single-stage osteotomy of the short ring finger metacarpal and immediate distraction and interposition of bone allograft with plate fixation.

the graft extraperiosteally to prevent resorption and provide the best chance for epiphyseal growth. They reported 36 toe phalangeal bone grafts in 20 children performed between the ages of 6 months and 13 years. With a mean follow-up of 2.4 years postoperatively, 24% of bone grafts overall showed epiphyseal closure, primarily related to the older age of the child at the time of surgery. When surgery was performed between 6 and 18 months of age, 91% of the epiphyses remained open and growth averaged 83% to 100% of the contralateral toe. When surgery was performed between 18 months and 5 years of age, 67% of the epiphyses remained open, but growth still averaged 80% to 100%. Finally, when surgery was performed after 5 years of age, only 50% of epiphyses remained open, but growth was still 90% of the contralateral phalanx.

Buck-Gramcko[6] reiterated the importance of harvesting the periosteum with the phalanx for the best results. He reported 69 nonvascularized toe phalangeal bone grafts in 46 children between 7 months and 17 years of age. The results were analyzed according to the child's age at the time of surgery. Group I consisted of children undergoing surgery up to 18 months of age, group II between 19 months and 4 years of age, and group III over 4 years of age. Epiphyses remained open in 65%, 27%, and 16%, respectively, with average growth of 3 mm, 3.5 mm, and 1.5 mm, respectively, in each group. There was no measurable growth in 15 toe phalangeal bone grafts (21%). A new secondary technique was introduced in four children in which an osteotomy was performed in the middle third of the toe phalangeal bone graft; distraction was applied, and an iliac crest

bone graft was inserted to produce a further increase in length of 8 to 12 mm.

Radocha and colleagues[7] reported 73 toe phalangeal bone grafts in 26 children with a mean follow-up of 42 months. The children were again grouped by their age at the time of surgery: younger than 12 months of age, 12 to 24 months of age, and older than 24 months of age. The epiphyses remained open in 94%, 70.5%, and 48% of children, respectively. This study showed a significant difference in expected growth when compared with Goldberg and Watson's results, with only 71% of the contralateral growth compared with 90% reported by Goldberg and Watson.

Cavallo and colleagues[8] demonstrated that better results could be obtained by harvesting the middle phalanx rather than the proximal phalanx. They reported 64 toe phalangeal bone grafts in 22 children—35 using the proximal phalanx and 29 using the middle phalanx. There was an average resorption of 0.7 mm using the proximal phalanx graft, whereas the middle phalanx bone graft had an average net growth of 0.8 mm, which was attributed to the intact cortical barrier of the middle phalanx.

Tonkin and colleagues[9] reported 21 nonvascularized toe phalangeal bone transfers in 13 children with transverse arrest and a mean follow-up of 7.4 years. Of the 18 surviving transfers, 4 continued to have open physes. The average length of the transferred phalanx was 75% compared with the contralateral toe phalanx. Of the 10 patients able to undergo functional testing, 5 used the transferred phalanx for complex tasks, 2 for simple tasks, and 3 for assist only. Most parents felt satisfied with the appearance of the hand but also felt there was no significant improvement.

Unglaub and colleagues[10] also emphasized the importance of early surgery and extraperiosteal harvesting and reported that epiphyses remained open in 79% overall. They analyzed their results according to the age of the children at the time of surgery: up to 18 months of age, 18 months to 4 years of age, and older than 4 years of age. The best results were seen in the group with ages between 18 months and 4 years. In most cases, there was only passive movement of the metacarpophalangeal joint, but 75% of the parents noted significant functional improvement.

Summary

Nonvascularized toe phalangeal bone grafts have been the main conventional surgical option for reconstruction of hypoplastic digits; however, the results have been inconsistent. The average length of a toe proximal phalanx graft is approximately 12 to 15 mm in a 1- to 2-year-old child. They can provide some modest lengthening of a hypoplastic digit and definitely provide stability to an empty skin envelope (**Fig. 4**). The likelihood that the transferred epiphyses remain open is optimized if the toe phalanx is harvested extraperiosteally and if the surgery is performed early before 1 to 1.5 years of age. Increased length of the hypoplastic digit may be achieved by secondary osteotomy, distraction, and bone grafting of the previously transferred toe phalangeal bone graft. With the success of microsurgical toe-to-hand transfers, the indications for nonvascularized toe phalangeal bone grafts are likely to decline.

DISTRACTION LENGTHENING

Lengthening a bone through callus distraction with or without secondary intercalary bone grafting is another conventional technique in the hand surgeon's armamentarium. The concept of lengthening bones by means of distraction was first introduced by Codivilla in 1905, when he described lengthening the lower extremities in congenital deficiencies. Matev applied this concept to the upper extremity in 1970 in three patients with previous thumb amputations who underwent osteotomy of the thumb metacarpal followed by gradual distraction.[11] Initially the osteotomy bone gap was allowed to consolidate spontaneously, but secondary bone grafting using autograft or allograft speeds up the consolidation. A complete osteotomy was originally described, but other surgeons have described distraction after corticotomy. Distraction was originally recommended at a rate of 1 mm/day, but slower rates

of 0.25 mm twice daily or four times daily have become more standard. Indications for distraction lengthening were initially for posttraumatic amputations but have evolved to include digital aplasia and hypoplasia.

Matev[12] described seven children ranging in age from 10 to 14 years in whom metacarpal lengthening was performed to reconstruct amputation stumps. Distraction lengthening lasted an average of 35 days and resulted in an increase in length of 2.5 to 3.8 cm, with an average increase in length of 88%. In all cases, there was no need for secondary interposition bone grafting because the metacarpals spontaneously consolidated. All lengthened digits had pinch strengths close or equal to that of the normal contralateral hand. There were no complications in any of the seven patients.

Kessler and colleagues[13] described 11 children with congenital abnormalities who underwent distraction lengthening of one or more metacarpals between 5 and 11 years of age; 2.5 to 4 cm of metacarpal length was achieved by distraction. A second-stage interposition bone graft was performed as soon as the distraction lengthening had finished to decrease the incidence of infection from the Kirschner wires and allow earlier union rather than waiting for the bone to consolidate spontaneously.

Smith and Gumley[14] described 24 patients who underwent distraction lengthening of 41 metacarpals, 30 of which were caused by congenital abnormalities, 3 of which were caused by premature epiphyseal closure, and 8 that resulted from traumatic thumb amputations. Patient ages ranged from 1 to 50 years, and total lengthening ranged from 1 to 4.5 cm, with the greatest increase seen in the posttraumatic group. In all groups, the patient and/or family members noted a marked increase in function, although in the group with congenital abnormalities, a valid comparison of preoperative and postoperative function was not performed.

Seitz and Froimson[15,16] reported 14 distraction lengthenings or "callostasis" for congenital anomalies and posttraumatic defects in eight patients with an age range from 2 to 66 years. Eleven proximal phalanges and three thumb metacarpals were lengthened at a rate of 1 mm/day divided into four 0.25-mm distractions of the lengthening device per day. Lengthening was started on postoperative day 5 for the children and postoperative day 7 for the adults. The authors reported an increase in length from 2.5 to 3.5 cm and increased function in all cases.

Netscher and Richards[17] described a child with symbrachydactyly born with a normal thumb but

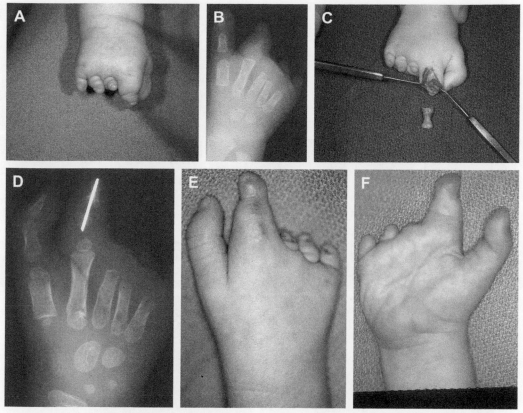

Fig. 4. (*A, B*) Symbrachydactyly of the right hand with a relatively normal thumb but hypoplastic fingers. (*C*) A nonvascularized toe phalangeal bone graft was harvested extraperiosteally from the second toe. (*D–F*) One year postoperatively, the nonvascularized toe phalangeal bone graft provided increased length and stability and improved pinch of the right index finger.

only a proximal phalanx for the index finger and nubbins for the ulnar three digits. The child initially underwent nonvascularized toe phalangeal bone grafting of the index, middle, ring, and small fingers followed by web space deepening. When the child's thumb outgrew the other digits, distraction lengthening of the ulnar four fingers was performed followed by iliac crest bone grafting of the ulnar three digits to achieve bony fusion. The small finger was lengthened 20 mm and the middle and ring fingers were lengthened 27 mm each.

Summary

Distraction lengthening of either a metacarpal or phalanx remains a powerful tool for reconstruction of a hypoplastic digit and may produce 1 to 4 cm of increased length. Children seem to tolerate the lengthening device well, and there are few reports of pain associated with distraction as long as the device is lengthened slowly. Bony union of the distraction gap is achieved more rapidly with

a second-stage interposition bone graft, however (**Fig. 5**).

MICROSURGICAL TOE-TO-HAND TRANSFERS

Advances in microsurgical techniques probably have made toe-to-hand transfers the emerging standard for the treatment of hypoplastic and aplastic digits. The first microsurgical toe-to-hand transfer for a congenital hand deformity was reported in 1978 by O'Brien and colleagues,[18] who described two children who underwent transfer of a great toe to reconstruct the thumb. Since then, microsurgical techniques have vastly improved, and current series report success rates of more than 95%.[19–30] Indications for toe-to-hand transfers include multiple missing digits at the metacarpophalangeal joint level or more proximally and multiple severely hypoplastic digits at the level of the proximal phalanges or proximal interphalangeal joints. Pollicization remains the standard procedure for reconstructing an absent thumb with four fingers, but if the thumb is absent

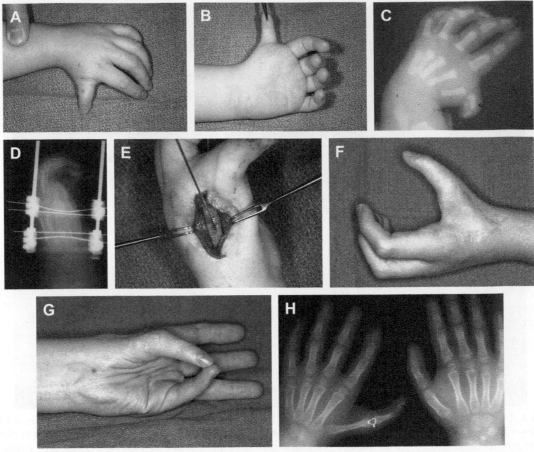

Fig. 5. (A–C) A 3-year-old boy with brachydactyly of his left thumb. The parents refused pollicization of the index finger. (D, E) Distraction lengthening of the thumb metacarpal was followed by interposition bone grafting at a second stage and release of the thumb-index finger web space with a full-thickness skin graft and an opposition tendon transfer using the flexor digitorum sublimis tendon from the ring finger. (F–H) Three years postoperatively, the reconstructed thumb demonstrated satisfactory length and opposition and was used for all activities.

because of congenital constriction ring syndrome and the metacarpal and thenar muscles are relatively normal, a toe-to-thumb transfer probably provides better results. The second toe is usually preferred for reconstruction of hypoplastic or aplastic fingers because the donor site in the foot is relatively inconspicuous and the second toe is positioned on the ulnar side of the hand, which allows grasp and pinch.

Timing of Surgery

The age of the child must be considered during preoperative planning. Benefits of early surgery include increased adaptation time before starting school, parental satisfaction, and growth potential; however, the recipient vessels and nerves must be present and large enough to allow microsurgical anastomoses. Gilbert[19] concluded that a vessel needs to be 1 mm or larger in diameter for optimal

results, but this is not always evident unless a preoperative angiogram is done. Kay and Wiberg[25] reported only one case out of 66 toe transfers (1.6%) in which the transfer had to be abandoned because adequate recipient nerves could not be identified. Surgical intervention should be performed before the child starts school because peers can be unforgiving in their criticism. Unilateral deficiencies may need to be treated earlier than bilateral deficiencies so that use of the normal hand does not cause neglect of the involved hand. Lister[21] reported microsurgical toe-to-hand transfers performed between 6 months and 1 year of age, but the senior author generally waits until 2 years of age.

Parents must be informed of the implications of this major procedure. They must understand a realistic potential outcome for function and appearance and must be able to accept the small probability for failure of the toe transfer, which

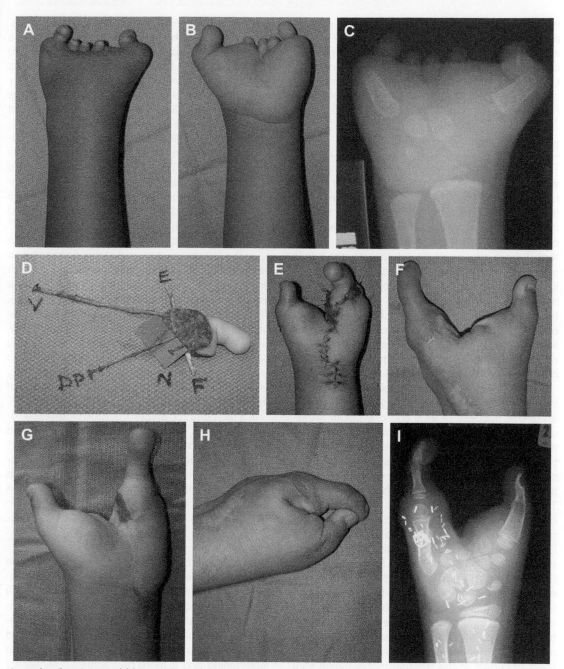

Fig. 6. (*A–C*) A 2-year-old boy with symbrachydactyly of his left hand with a hypoplastic thumb and essentially nubbins representing the fingers. The radiograph shows only metacarpals to the thumb and small finger and remnants of distal phalanges in the thumb and small finger. (*D, E*) Second toe transfer on to the small finger metacarpal. In the same operation, part of the second toe metatarsal was used as a conventional bone graft to stabilize and lengthen the left thumb. (*F–H*) Three years postoperatively, the child had excellent pinch and grasp between the second toe transfer and the lengthened thumb. (*I*) The radiograph shows consolidation of the metatarsal bone graft between the metacarpal and the remnant of the distal phalanx of the thumb.

would leave the child with the same hand without any increase in function and a missing toe. Parents also must consider the defect in the donor foot, but parents do not usually report any difficulty in balance or ambulation after a toe transfer, and most surgeons consider the donor morbidity of harvesting a second toe to be minimal.

Results

The initial descriptions of toe-to-hand transfers were case reports, but since then, larger series have reported success rates to be more than 96% with dramatically improved function, sensation, and growth. Buck-Gramcko[22] described operations in which 26 second toes were transferred from the contralateral foot to the ulnar aspect of the hand with "satisfactory" results but limited active range of motion of the transferred toe. Shvedovchenko[23] reported 103 toe-to-hand transfers in 66 children aged 3 to 14 years with posttraumatic deformities and congenital anomalies. The authors noted acceptable esthetic results, but three transfers required secondary distraction lengthening for increased length.

Vilkki[24] reported 18 microsurgical toe transfers in children ranging from 2 to 12 years of age with an overall success of 94% and one failure attributed to anesthesia complications. Five of the remaining 17 transfers required early re-exploration to revise the microsurgical anastomoses. Fifteen children were considered to have increased hand function, but growth could not be assessed fully. There was absolutely no donor site morbidity in any of the children. Kay and colleagues[25,26] reported the largest study to date of pediatric toe-to-hand transfers with complete survival of 135 toe transfers. Initially there was a 6% re-exploration rate, which decreased to 2% with increasing experience. Average two-point discrimination was 4 mm, and 20% of children required secondary surgeries, including tenolysis or tendon transfers in an attempt to improve active range of motion. The authors reported that the most movement occurred at the metacarpophalangeal joint and there was increased functionality in the hand.

Van Holder and colleagues[27] reported 14 children who underwent staged double second toe transfers. The first toe transfer was performed at an average age of 3 years, 8 months, with an average of 12 months between the two toe transfers. Mean total active flexion was 80° with a mean extension lag of 20°, but all patients required secondary operations, including tenolysis, repair of tendon rupture, web space deepening, secondary tendon grafting or transfer, opponensplasty, metacarpal osteotomy, and ligament reconstruction. Foucher and colleagues[28] reported 65 toe-to-hand transfers with an average follow-up of 5.2 years. They had no failures if two arteries were anastomosed to the transferred toe, but two failures occurred if only one artery was anastomosed. The mean total active range of motion was 38°, and the mean two-point discrimination was 5 mm.

Jones and colleagues[29] reported 82 toe-to-hand transfers in 68 children with congenital hand anomalies. Two toe transfers (2.4%) failed and 7 (8.5%) required re-exploration of the microsurgical anastomoses. All children regained protective sensation, and all but 2 developed improved hand function. Tu and colleagues[30] concluded that toe-to-thumb transfer was an acceptable treatment for radial deficiencies as an alternative to pollization. They reported on 11 children aged 18 months to 6 years who underwent toe transfers to reconstruct a hypoplastic thumb. The success rate was 90.9%, and 1 patient underwent immediate re-exploration for venous occlusion. The mean total active range of motion was 60°, and the mean total passive range of motion was 117°. Sensation was regained in all toe transfers, with an average two-point discrimination of 4.2 mm. There was no donor site morbidity.

In a radiographic analysis of growth after toe-to-hand transfers, Chang and Jones[31] demonstrated that the epiphyses remained open; there was increasing serial growth of the toe transfer compared with preoperative radiographs, and serial growth of the toe transfer was exactly the same as the contralateral toe.

SUMMARY

Microsurgical toe-to-hand transfer is perhaps the most powerful and rewarding technique for reconstruction of severe hypoplasia and aplasia of the digits. The second toe is approximately 5 cm long in a 2-year-old child and provides an immediate and much larger increase in length compared with toe phalangeal bone grafting or distraction lengthening and a more guaranteed potential for serial growth. It also provides sensation and some limited range of motion. The operation requires meticulous microsurgical skills, and sometimes it is difficult to convince parents to consider a toe transfer, but this procedure has the greatest potential to create functional grasp and pinch in a hypoplasic digit or hand (**Fig. 6**).

REFERENCES

1. Flatt AE. The care of congenital hand anomalies. St. Louis (MO): Quality Medical; 1994.

2. Swanson AB. A classification for congenital limb malformation. J Hand Surg 1976;1:8–22.

3. Blauth W, Gekeler J. Morphology and classification of symbrachydactylia. Hand 1971;3:123–8.

4. Jones NF. Nonvascularized toe phalangeal bone grafts for congenital anomalies of the hand. J Am Soc Surg Hand 2004;4:27–34.

5. Goldberg NH, Watson HK. Composite toe (phalanx and epiphyses) transfers and reconstruction of the aphalangic hand. J Hand Surg [Am] 1982;7:454–9.

6. Buck-Gramcko D. The role of non-vascularized toe phalanx transplantation. Hand Clin 1990;6:642–59.

7. Radocha RF, Netscher D, Kleiner HE. Toe phalangeal grafts in congenital hand anomalies. J Hand Surg 1993;18A:833–41.

8. Cavallo AV, Smith PJ, Morley S, et al. Non-vascularized free toe phalanx transfers in congenital hand deformities: the Great Ormond Street experience. J Hand Surg [Br] 2003;6:520–7.

9. Tonkin MA, Deva AK, Filan SL. Long term follow-up of composite non-vascularized toe phalanx transfers for aphalangia. J Hand Surg [Br] 2005;30:452–8.

10. Unglaub F, Lanz U, Hahn P. Outcome analysis, including patient and parental satisfaction, regarding nonvascularized free toe phalanx transfer in congenital hand deformities. Ann Plast Surg 2006;56:87–92.

11. Matev IB. Thumb reconstruction after amputation at the metacarpophalangeal joint by bone lengthening. J Bone Joint Surg 1970;52A:957–65.

12. Matev IB. Thumb reconstruction in children through metacarpal lengthening. Plast Reconstr Surg 1979;64:665–9.

13. Kessler I, Baruch A, Hecht O. Experience with distraction lengthening of digital rays in congenital anomalies. J Hand Surg 1977;2:394–401.

14. Smith RJ, Gumley G. Metacarpal distraction lengthening. Hand Clin 1985;1:417–29.

15. Seitz WH, Froimson AL. Digital lengthening using the callotasis technique. Orthopedics 1995;18:129–38.

16. Seitz WH, Froimson AL. Callotasis lengthening in the upper extremity: indications, techniques, and pitfalls. J Hand Surg [Am] 1991;16:932–9.

17. Netscher DT, Richards WT. Rational treatment for multiple digit congenital absence: case report of nonvascularized toe phalangeal transfers and distraction lengthening for symbrachydactyly. Ann Plast Surg 2006;56:211–5.

18. O'Brien BM, Black MJM, Morrison WA, et al. Microvascular great toe transfer for congenital absence of the thumb. Hand 1978;10:113–24.

19. Gilbert A. Toe transfers for congenital hand defects. J Hand Surg [Am] 1982;7:118–24.

20. Gilbert A. Reconstruction of congenital hand defects with microvascular toe transfers. Hand Clin 1985;1:351–60.

21. Lister G. Microsurgical transfer of the second toe for congenital deficiency of the thumb. Plast Reconstr Surg 1988;82:658–65.

22. Buck-Gramcko D. Progress in the treatment of congenital malformations of the hand. World J Surg 1990;14:715–24.

23. Shvedovchenko IV. Toe-to-hand transfers in children. Ann Plast Surg 1993;3:251–4.

24. Vilkki S. Advances in microsurgical reconstruction of the congenitally adactylous hand. Clin Orthop Relat Res 1995;314:45–8.

25. Kay SP, Wiberg M. Toe to hand transfer in children. Part 1. Technical aspects. J Hand Surg [Br] 1996;21:723–34.

26. Kay S, McGuiness C. Microsurgical reconstruction in abnormalities of children's hands. Hand Clin 1999;15:563–83.

27. Van Holder C, Giele H, Gilbert A. Double second toe transfer in congenital hand anomalies. J Hand Surg [Br] 1996;24:471–5.

28. Foucher G, Medina J, Navarro R, et al. Toe transfer in congenital hand malformations. J Reconstr Microsurg 2001;17:1–7.

29. Jones NF, Hansen SL, Bates SJ. Toe-to-hand transfers for congenital anomalies of the hand. Hand Clin 2007;23:129–36.

30. Tu Y-K, Yeh W-L, Sananpanich K, et al. Microsurgical second toe-metatarsal bone transfer for reconstructing congenital radial deficiency with hypoplastic thumb. J Reconstr Microsurg 2004;20:215–25.

31. Chang J, Jones NF. Radiographic analysis of growth in pediatric microsurgical toe-to-hand transfers. Plast Reconstr Surg 2002;109:576–82.

Constriction Band Syndrome

Kenji Kawamura, MD, PhD[a], Kevin C. Chung, MD[b],*

KEYWORDS

- Constriction band syndrome • Malformation
- Congenital anomaly • Hand • Treatment

Constriction band syndrome is a relatively rare condition in which fetal parts become entangled in the amniotic membrane, leading to deformation, malformation, and amputation. Many terms have been used for this complex anomaly, including constriction band syndrome,[1] amniotic band syndrome,[2] congenital annular constrictions,[3] congenital ring constrictions,[4] and intrauterine amputation.[5] The overabundance of synonyms for constriction band syndrome is caused by confusion regarding its etiology. Recent reports revealed that constriction band syndrome or amniotic band syndrome might be the most frequently used term to describe this complex congenital anomaly.[6–11] Although capricious manifestations do occur in constriction band syndrome, several characteristic features are relatively consistent findings. Distal ring constrictions, intrauterine amputations, and acrosyndactyly are the most common findings in this syndrome and are typically seen in the distal aspect of extremities.[8,9] Multiple extremity involvement is usually expressed, with an average of three affected extremity parts.[9] Deformations affecting the upper extremities are disabling and pose a treatment challenge for hand surgeons because of the unique presentations in each individual.[12]

EPIDEMIOLOGY AND ETIOLOGY

The reported incidence of constriction band syndrome varies from 1/1,200 to 1/15,000 live births.[4,9,13,14] No distinct sex predilection has been determined. Nearly 60% of the documented cases have some sort of abnormal gestation history.[9] Prenatal risk factors associated with constriction band syndrome include: prematurity (<37 weeks); low birth weight (<2,500 g); maternal drug exposure; and maternal illness or trauma during pregnancy. Attempted abortion in the first trimester is also a highly associated risk factor. No autosomal inheritance pattern has been identified, and maternal prenatal infection does not appear to be an associated feature.

Although the etiology of constriction band syndrome remains controversial, there are two main theories that may explain the development of this syndrome. The first is the intrinsic theory, proposed by Streeter in 1930,[5] which suggests that constriction band syndrome represents an inherent development defect in embryogenesis. In this theory, the bands arise from an endogenous defect in germ plasm differentiation that causes the limb to become necrotic and form fibrous bands. Some authors who support Streeter's intrinsic theory have expanded on it by suggesting teratogenic insult, viral infection, or vascular disruption as the cause of the malformations in constriction band syndrome. In 1961, Patterson[15] explained the etiology of the syndrome as a primary failure of the development of the subcutaneous tissue during the morphogenetic period. Van Allen and coworkers[16] suggested that amputations and constriction rings may be due to vascular disturbances. Lockwood and coworkers[17] reviewed 14 cases of twin gestations associated with constriction band syndrome and reported that the disorder was more common in monozygotic twinning, thereby supporting a teratogenic cause.

Supported in part by a Midcareer Investigator Award in Patient-Oriented Research (K24 AR053120) from the National Institute of Arthritis and Musculoskeletal and Skin Diseases (to Kevin C. Chung).

[a] Department of Orthopaedic Surgery, Nara Medical University, 840 Shijyo-cho, Kashihara, Nara 634-8522, Japan

[b] Section of Plastic Surgery, Department of Surgery, University of Michigan Medical School, 2130 Taubman Center, 1500 E. Medical Center Drive, Ann Arbor, MI 48109-0340, USA

* Corresponding author.

E-mail address: kecchung@umich.edu (K.C. Chung).

Hand Clin 25 (2009) 257–264

doi:10.1016/j.hcl.2008.10.007

An alternative view for the etiology of constriction band syndrome was described by Torpin in 1965.[18] He proposed an extrinsic theory, in which early amnion rupture forms adherent bands that constrict, entangle, and amputate limbs. As the amnion ruptures, it slips off the chorion to form the detaching mesoblastic fibrous strands. These strands subsequently become entangled around the digits or limbs. The denuded chorion then absorbs the amniotic fluid and causes a temporary oligohydramnios or compressive environment. Torpin's extrinsic theory is supported by the findings of many authors. Kino[1] successfully produced acrosyndactyly in animal experiments involving amniotic sac puncture, and concluded that this anomaly was due to hemorrhage from the marginal blood sinuses of the digital rays in already developed or developing limb buds. Higginbottom and coworkers[19] suggested that early amniotic rupture leads to severely affected infants who are frequently absorbed or stillborn, whereas later amniotic rupture primarily results in limb involvement. Foulkes and Reinker[9] conjectured that amniotic disruption before 7 weeks of gestation is more likely to produce limb reduction, polysyndactyly, and syndactyly secondary to interference with segmentation, whereas later amniotic rupture yields mechanical deformation of amniotic bands, clubfoot, distal hypoplasia, lymphedema, and intrauterine amputations. The occurrence of asymmetric deformities with nonembryologic distributions also supports Torpin's extrinsic theory.

Although there has been much debate over the cause of constriction band syndrome, the majority of contemporary authors have described Torpin's extrinsic theory as the most appropriate explanation for the entire clinical spectrum of constriction band syndrome.[1,9,10,13,19,20]

CLINICAL PRESENTATION

The clinical manifestations are predominantly distal deformities such as constriction of limbs and fingers, syndactyly, acrosyndactyly (fenestrated syndactyly), phalangeal hypoplasia, and amputation of limbs and fingers.[8,9] Multiple malformations such as clubfoot (30% of patients), leg length discrepancies (24%), other bone anomalies (12%), special craniofacial defects such as cleft lip and palate (8%), visceral and body wall defects, and anencephaly (5%) have been detected in 70% of infants with the disorder.[8,9,21,22] Owing to the fact that no two cases with this syndrome are exactly alike, only some of the above-mentioned anomalies are present in each individual case.

The clinical presentation in the hand varies from slight indentations on the affected part to distal atrophy, lymphedema, acrosyndactyly, and amputation (**Fig. 1**). From the hand surgeon's perspective, the most important aspect is that the structures of the hand proximal to the constriction band are normal. If the ring constriction is severe, the veins, arteries, lymphatics, and nerves may be compromised.[21] Neurologic impairment is usually attributed to axonotmesis or neurotmesis. This may be caused by direct pressure from the constriction band or attributable to compartment syndrome distal to the band in infants with rapidly progressive swelling. Distal digits are typically malformed owing to phalangeal hypoplasia or terminal amputation. Acrosyndactyly is frequently associated with distal amputation.[23] This type of syndactyly involves binding of adjacent digits in a lassoed appearance. If acrosyndactyly is present, it is invariably associated with a proximal interdigital sinus or cleft that communicates from the dorsal side to the volar side (**Fig. 2**). Cutaneous syndactyly does not usually involve underlying bony fusion.

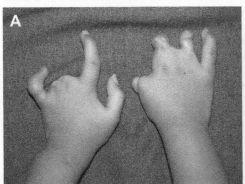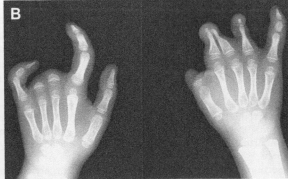

Fig. 1. A 4-year-old boy with constriction band syndrome. (*A*) Right hand showing amputation of the thumb and ring finger and acrosyndactyly of the index and long fingers, with left hand showing amputation of the long and ring fingers, angulated index and little fingers, and lymphedema of the little finger. (*B*) Radiograph of the same patient showing acrosyndactyly of right index and long fingers associated with distal amputations.

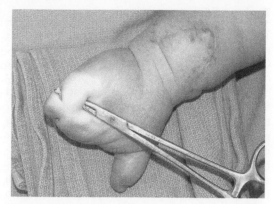

Fig. 2. Acrosyndactyly with a probe in the sinus tract.

There is a predilection for the hand as the site of involvement.[7,9] The central digits are often involved, whereas the frequency and severity of thumb involvement are minimal, even when all the fingers are severely affected. Foulkes and Reinker[9] reported that, among 93 affected hands, the ring finger was most frequently involved (89.2%) followed by the long (86%), index (71%), and little (51.6%) fingers. The incidence of thumb involvement was only 21.5%. Several reasons have been proposed for the lack of thumb involvement.[1,7,11] First, with fetal hand positioning, with either outstretched fingers or a clenched thumb in the palm, the thumb is protected by the other fingers. Second, the developmental difference of each digital ray may have correlation with the predilection. Thumb development precedes that of the central digits, and it is assumed that constriction band syndrome occurs at the later stage of limb development because the involved parts are relatively well developed—and delivery of a well-developed amputated extremity has been reported. Third, anatomic differences should be considered. The thumb and little finger have independent blood supplies from separate digital vessels. If the etiology of constriction band syndrome is due to hemorrhage within the limb bud, as suggested by Kino,[1] this anatomic difference may play an important role in the predilection for site involvement.

DIAGNOSIS

Ultrasonographic analysis allows prenatal detection of constriction band syndrome by visualization of amniotic bands attached to the fetus.[24] In the first trimester, it is extremely difficult to detect the syndrome, especially if the amniotic bands are limited to the extremities. In the second and third trimesters, it is relatively easy to detect the major anomalies of the syndrome by their characteristic features and restriction of fetal movements.[25] Radiography may reveal severe skeletal defects such as absent cranial ossification, severe limb deformities, or spinal deformities.[13] As the more serious manifestations of the condition are outside the limbs, in the head, neck, and trunk, neonatal diagnosis is frequently difficult and is accurately accomplished in only 29%–50% of cases in the absence of specialized genetic consultation.[2,19] Only 13% of constriction band syndrome cases with severe craniofacial deformities have been reported to be correctly diagnosed.[13] The craniofacial deformities present in constriction band syndrome are typically bizarre and frequently nonembryologic in location. As many as one in 20 anencephalic babies may have constriction band syndrome.[19] The incorrect diagnosis is usually that of the most prominent anomaly observed. The presence of fibrous bands at constriction points is helpful in the diagnosis.

For isolated extremities, the important differential diagnoses of constriction band syndrome include symbrachydactyly and transverse deficiency. Symbrachydactyly usually affects the entire hand, and the patient typically has a small hand with simple syndactyly. Bilateral cases of symbrachydactyly are rare, ranging from 1.6%–10%,[12] whereas multiple areas in more than one extremity are usually involved in constriction band syndrome.[9] The defect of symbrachydactyly is believed to be mesodermal, which explains the presence of distal finger ectodermal structures such as pulp, nail fold, and nail. Symbrachydactyly may occur with Poland syndrome. Ogino and Saitou[26] performed a detailed comparison of constriction band syndrome and transverse deficiency. Transverse deficiency is more often unilateral, whereas constriction band syndrome is bilateral. Transverse deficiency tends to be more proximal, and rudimentary fingernails are common. Bone hypoplasia may be found in neighboring fingers or proximally in the limb in transverse deficiency. Amputations in constriction band syndrome tend to have tapering bone stumps, whereas transverse deficiencies more often take the form of disarticulations.

CLASSIFICATION

Several classification systems of the limb lesions in constriction band syndrome have been devised, but they add little to the clinical understanding because constriction band syndrome is a complex collection of asymmetric congenital anomalies, in which no two cases are exactly alike. The most widely used classification system was proposed by Patterson,[15] and is based on the severity of the syndrome (**Box 1**). There are four categories in Patterson's classification, namely: simple constriction rings, constriction rings associated with deformity of the distal part with or without lymphedema, constriction rings associated with acrosyndactyly, and intrauterine amputation. In addition, Patterson further divided the constriction rings associated with acrosyndactyly into three types: type I, conjoined fingertips with well-formed webs of the proper depth; type II, the tips of the digits are joined, but web formation is not complete; and type III, joined tips, sinus tracts between digits, and absent webs.

TREATMENT

Treatment of constriction band syndrome must be individualized, and ranges from cosmetic repair to emergency limb-sparing band release. Shallow bands may require no operative treatment unless they interfere with circulation or lymphatic drainage. Cosmetic repair of shallow bands without lymphedema may be done electively. Deep bands require release of the constriction bands by circumferential Z-plasty or W-plasty. In cases with severe ischemia, which may lead to osteomyelitis, amputation of the distal part may be considered. On-top plasty (partial digital transfer), toe-to-hand transfer, bone lengthening procedures, and pollicization procedures have been performed to restore function in cases with digital hypoplasia and amputation. In patients with acrosyndactyly, separation of digits and web reconstruction are required. Current improvements in prenatal diagnosis and fetoscopic surgical techniques may eventually allow in utero treatment of constriction band syndrome.[25,27]

Box 1
Patterson's classification of constriction band syndrome

1. Simple constriction rings
2. Constriction rings associated with the deformity of the distal part, with or without lymphedema
3. Constriction rings associated with acrosyndactyly
   Type I: conjoined fingertips with well-formed webs of the proper depth
   Type II: the tips of the digits are joined, but web formation is not complete
   Type III: joined tips, sinus tracts between digits, and absent webs
4. Intrauterine amputation

Timing of Surgery

The timing of surgery is determined by the disease severity and predicted skeletal growth. Constriction bands with severe distal lymphedema, cyanosis, and circulatory problems may progress quickly to irreversible ischemia and subsequent ulceration or infection. In such patients, urgent release of the bands should be performed within a few days after birth. In other cases, removal of the constriction bands is accomplished by single or two-stage release, usually beginning at 3 months of age. Some authors advocate a two-stage procedure to avoid vascular interruption to the distal segment.[21] Only 50% of the band is released at a time, and once the cutaneous circulation has been reestablished across the scar, the remaining 50% of the band can be released safely. An interval of 6–12 weeks between the procedures is advised.[11] Most experts recommend single release for superficial bands and two-stage release for deep bands.[28,29] In patients with acrosyndactyly, surgery is recommended between the ages of 6 months and 1 year to allow for proper longitudinal bone growth.

Release of Constriction Bands

Regardless of the technique used for release of the constriction band, all authors agree that the constriction band should be excised and discarded, and not used as part of the reconstructive flap (**Fig. 3**). The contracted portions of the band remain deformed during transposition and can add to the residual defect. Other surgical considerations include the preservation of at least one or two large subcutaneous veins along with the neurovascular bundle to prevent postoperative distal venous congestion. In cases with deep dorsal bands, there is often a paucity of dorsal veins, and two-stage release should be considered.

Traditionally, release of constriction bands has been performed by serial Z-plasties of skin following excision of the fibrotic constriction band. This traditional technique is not effective for eliminating the contour deformity in severe cases. The sandglass deformity, which results from subcutaneous tissue deficiency under the constriction band, persists after using the traditional technique. In 1991, Upton and Tan[30] described a new technique for constriction band release to prevent recurrent contour deformities. After excision of the constriction band and debulking of excess adipose tissue, the mobilized subcutaneous adipose flap is advanced into the defect as a separate layer, with thin Z-plasties transposed separately (**Fig. 4**).

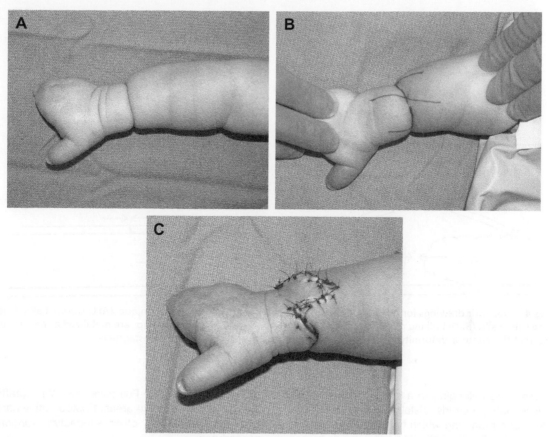

Fig. 3. (*A*) Ring constriction of right distal forearm. (*B*) The design of Z-plasties is shown. (*C*) Appearance after excision of the groove and repair with Z-plasties.

Z-plasties are positioned along the side of the digit with a straight-line closure dorsally to minimize visible scarring. Many authors have reported successful results using Upton's technique for the treatment of constriction bands.[11,12,31] However, in cases with a broad constriction band, a cross-finger flap may be used to replace the deficient area. If multiple digits are involved, a large flap such as a groin flap may be considered. As with every case of constriction bands, the treatment should be tailored to the individual.

Surgery for Acrosyndactyly

Acrosyndactyly is a condition in which two or more fingers are fused at their terminal portions with proximal epithelial lined clefts or sinuses between the fingers.[23] The goals of surgery for acrosyndactyly are to separate the fingers and create a web space to provide the best functional results (**Fig. 5**). Surgical planning should be guided by the dictum that the number of fingers is not as

important as their spacing, length, bulk, stability, and control.[11] Standard syndactyly techniques are used as much as possible. In general, the fingers are separated with carefully planned zigzag incisions, and a broad commissural space is created with a dorsal skin flap. Surgery should only be performed on one side of a finger at a time. Most patients with acrosyndactyly associated with constriction band syndrome have type III defects (joined tips, sinus tracts between digits and absent web) according to Patterson's classification. If the sinus tract is inadequate to function as a web space because of its distal location and narrow space, it can be excised and may be used as a skin graft. Occassionally, the sinus tract may contain adequate skin at its base; this skin can be retained to serve as the web space skin. Finger separation is easiest when performed in the proximal to distal direction. However, standard syndactyly separation techniques occasionally cannot be used distally because the fingers distal to the point of fusion may not be clearly

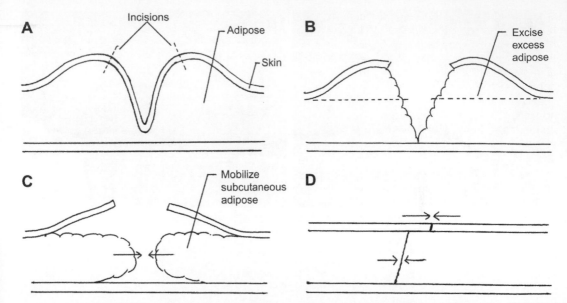

Fig. 4. Schematic drawings for releasing of the constriction band with Upton's technique. (*A*) Excision of all skin in the side walls. (*B*) Debulking of excess adipose tissue. (*C*) Subcutaneous adipose flaps are mobilized as needed to correct the contour deformity. (*D*) Skin and subcutaneous closures are preferably staggered.

defined as belonging to a specific finger. As the dissection proceeds distally, a decision should be made regarding which fingertip goes to which finger. An allocation should be then made by considering the survivability of the distal part as well as the resulting length and stability. Preservation of the distal tips is preferred over amputation because the tips may contain phalangeal buds that can be associated with articular spaces. Osteotomies can be performed to straighten severely angulated fingers. Every effort is made to preserve digital length, which can be reconstructed when

the child is larger. Full-thickness skin grafts are used to cover bare areas. Postoperative care is the same as for other syndactyly surgical procedures.

Reconstruction for Digital Hypoplasia and Amputation

Many procedures have been described for the treatment of digital hypoplasia and amputation associated with constriction band syndrome, including on-top plasty, toe-to-hand transfer, web

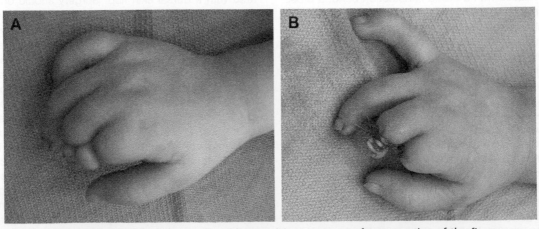

Fig. 5. (*A*) Acrosyndactyly of the index and long fingers. (*B*) Appearance after separation of the fingers.

space deepening, pollicization procedures, and bone lengthening procedures.[32,33] Management is aimed primarily at restoring basic hand function, specifically power grasp and precision pinch, and secondarily at improving the cosmetic appearance, which is inevitably going to be impaired. If the function of the hand is acceptable, no treatment may be a reasonable alternative.[11] As described previously, the thumb is preserved in most patients with constriction band syndrome, and thus treatment is often directed toward improving the functions of the remaining fingers. The structures proximal to the level of amputation are normal, making toe-to-hand transfer an attractive consideration. Toe-to-hand transfer is primarily performed at the ulnar digits to provide a pincer action. Limited mobility of the transferred toe allows the patient to use it as an ulnar post.[12] Metacarpal lengthening is also a useful and reliable procedure for amputated fingers to achieve functional and esthetic improvements.[32] Gradual metacarpal lengthening can be combined with bone grafting, or callus distraction may be performed without bone grafting. This procedure is usually reserved for patients older than 8 years, in whom the success rate is significantly higher than those in infant and toddlers.[34] Single-stage lengthening should be avoided because of frequently encountered complications, including collapse of the grafted bone, nonunion, and malunion.[32] On-top plasty is recommended when the index metacarpal is removed to provide a deep first web space in cases with absence of multiple digits. On-top plasty can be performed by transfer of a partially amputated index or ring finger to the "top" of an amputated long finger. Although the usual application of on-top plasty is to build on a thumb stump using the index metacarpal when the index finger is also missing, lengthening of the long finger can also be performed by this procedure for cases with an intact thumb and the absence of multiple digits. This partial digital transfer can both lengthen the digit and deepen the first web space when combined with index metacarpal shortening. During this procedure, care must be taken to avoid circulatory disturbance of the transposed index (or ring) stump because the neurovascular structures supplying the index (or ring) stump are short and have little capacity for mobilization. When the thumb is the only digit involved, index finger pollicization or thumb lengthening procedures can be performed. Toe-to-hand transfer is another option to reconstruct a deficient thumb. Absence of a thumb at the metacarpophalangeal joint level is a strong indication for toe-to-hand transfer.

SUMMARY

Constriction band syndrome is an uncommon congenital abnormality with multiple disfiguring and disabling manifestations. Early amnion rupture with subsequent entanglement of fetal parts by amniotic strands is the current primary theory for the development of this syndrome. Management of constriction band syndrome is focused on improving function and development while providing a more acceptable esthetic appearance. The treatment should be tailored to the individual. Timing of repair and surgical planning are important to provide the best functional results for affected hands.

REFERENCES

1. Kino Y. Clinical and experimental studies of the congenital constriction band syndrome, with an emphasis on its etiology. J Bone Joint Surg Am 1975;57(5): 636–43.
2. Ossipoff V, Hall BD. Etiologic factors in the amniotic band syndrome: a study of 24 patients. Birth Defects Orig Artic Ser 1977;13(3):117–32.
3. Isacsohn M, Aboulafia Y, Horowits B, et al. Congenital annular constrictions due to amniotic bands. Acta Obstet Gynecol Scand 1976;55(2):179–82.
4. Baker CJ, Rudolph AJ. Congenital ring constrictions and intrauterine amputations. Am J Dis Child 1971; 121(5):393–400.
5. Streeter GL. Focal deficiencies in fetal tissues and their relation to intrauterine amputation. Contrib Embryol 1930;22:1–44.
6. Miura T. Congenital constriction band syndrome. J Hand Surg [Am] 1984;9(1):82–8.
7. Tada K, Yonenobu K, Swanson AB. Congenital constriction band syndrome. J Pediatr Orthop 1984; 4(6):726–30.
8. Askins G, Ger E. Congenital constriction band syndrome. J Pediatr Orthop 1988;8(4):461–6.
9. Foulkes GD, Reinker K. Congenital constriction band syndrome: a seventy-year experience. J Pediatr Orthop 1994;14(2):242–8.
10. Woods T, Romansky N. Congenital constriction band syndrome. J Am Podiatr Med Assoc 1995;85(6):310–4.
11. Wiedrich TA. Congenital constriction band syndrome. Hand Clin 1998;14(1):29–38.
12. Moran SL, Jensen M, Bravo C. Amniotic band syndrome of the upper extremity: diagnosis and management. J Am Acad Orthop Surg 2007;15(7):397–407.
13. Seeds JW, Cefalo RC, Herbert WN. Amniotic band syndrome. Am J Obstet Gynecol 1982;144(3):243–8.
14. Fischer PM, Biddinger P, Drobnes WE. The amniotic band syndrome. Am Fam Physician 1983;27(2): 201–3.
15. Patterson TJ. Congenital ring-constrictions. Br J Plast Surg 1961;14:1–31.

16. Van Allen MI, Curry C, Walden CE, et al. Limb-body wall complex: II. Limb and spine defects. Am J Med Genet 1987;28(3):549–65.

17. Lockwood C, Ghidini A, Romero R, et al. Amniotic band syndrome: reevaluation of its pathogenesis. Am J Obstet Gynecol 1989;160(5):1030–3.

18. Torpin R. Amniochorionic mesoblastic fibrous strings and amniotic bands: associated constricting fetal malformations or fetal death. Am J Obstet Gynecol 1965;91:65–75.

19. Higginbottom MC, Jones KL, Hall BD, et al. The amniotic band disruption complex: timing of amniotic rupture and variable spectra of consequent defects. J Pediatr 1979;95(4):544–9.

20. Walter JH Jr, Goss LS, Lazzara AT. Amniotic band syndrome. J Foot Ankle Surg 1998;37(4):325–33.

21. Moses JM, Flatt AE, Cooper RR. Annular constricting bands. J Bone Joint Surg Am 1979;61(4):562–5.

22. de Pablo A, Calb I, Jaimovich L. Congenital constriction bands: amniotic band syndrome. J Am Acad Dermatol 1995;32(3):528–9.

23. Walsh RJ. Acrosyndactyly. A study of twenty-seven patients. Clin Orthop Relat Res 1970;71:99–111.

24. Mahony BS, Filly RA, Callen PW, et al. The amniotic band syndrome: antenatal sonographic diagnosis and potential pitfalls. Am J Obstet Gynecol 1985;152(1):63–8.

25. Burton DJ, Filly RA. Sonographic diagnosis of the amniotic band syndrome. AJR Am J Roentgenol 1991;156(3):555–8.

26. Ogino T, Saitou Y. Congenital constriction band syndrome and transverse deficiency. J Hand Surg [Br] 1987;12(3):343–8.

27. Ronderos-Dumit D, Briceno F, Navarro H, et al. Endoscopic release of limb constriction rings in utero. Fetal Diagn Ther 2006;21(3):255–8.

28. Hall EJ, Johnson-Giebink R, Vasconez LO. Management of the ring constriction syndrome: a reappraisal. Plast Reconstr Surg 1982;69(3):532–6.

29. Di Meo L, Mercer DH. Single-stage correction of constriction ring syndrome. Ann Plast Surg 1987;19(5):469–74.

30. Upton J, Tan C. Correction of constriction rings. J Hand Surg [Am] 1991;16(5):947–53.

31. Chung KC, Kim SE. Correction of constriction ring. In: Chung KC, editor. Operative techniques: hand and wrist surgery, 1st edition. Philadelphia: Saunders/Elsevier; 2007. p. 837–46.

32. Ogino T, Kato H, Ishii S, et al. Digital lengthening in congenital hand deformities. J Hand Surg [Br] 1994;19(1):120–9.

33. Papadogeorgou EV, Soucacos PN. Treatment alternatives of congenital hand differences with thumb hypoplasia involvement. Microsurgery 2008;28(2):121–30.

34. Matev IB. Thumb reconstruction through metacarpal bone lengthening. J Hand Surg [Am] 1980;5(5):482–7.

Generalized Skeletal Abnormalities

Andrew J. Watt, MD[a], Kevin C. Chung, MD[b],*

KEYWORDS
- Congenital trigger thumb
- Clasped thumb • Achondroplasia
- Madelung deformity • Congenital hand

The upper extremity is complex and its function relies on the precise arrangement of bone, cartilage, muscle, tendon, nerve and vascular structures acting in concord. This structure is, in turn, reliant upon the highly orchestrated temporal and spatial development, coordinated by molecular signaling and complex cellular interactions. This coordinated process allows undifferentiated mesenchyme and ectoderm to develop into the complex human limb. Given this complexity, it is not surprising that limb and hand abnormalities are among the most common congenital anomalies.

Congenital deformities affect 1% to 2% of all newborns and 10% of these deformities involve the upper extremity.[1,2] Congenital limb anomalies are classified according to the embryonic failure that underlies their clinical presentation. The most widely accepted classification, proposed by Frantz and O'Rahilly[3,4] and modified by Swanson, divides these anomalies into one of seven categories of embryologic failure: failure of formation of parts, failure of differentiation, duplication, overgrowth, undergrowth, congenital constriction band syndrome, and generalized skeletal abnormalities. The category of generalized skeletal anomalies is often applied for disorders that cannot be discretely categorized into one of the other six classes of embryologic failure. This article describes Swanson's broad category of generalized skeletal abnormalities, focusing on anomalies that are commonly seen in practice, including congenital trigger finger, congenital clasped thumb, and Madelung's deformity, as well as skeletal hand deformities that are characteristic of a generalized bone and connective tissue disorders, including achondroplasia and Marfan syndrome.

CONGENITAL FLEXION DEFORMITIES OF THE THUMB

The thumb plays a unique role in hand function. The degrees of freedom in flexion, extension, circumduction, and opposition of the thumb allow the hand to perform eloquent tasks while its strength imparts powerful grip. Thumb function develops gradually over the first year of life. Throughout the first four months of life, the thumb is characteristically held in a flexed, adducted position within the palm of the hand and is only intermittently extended. Thumb extension progresses around four months and ultimately culminates in the highly coordinated fine pinch grasp around one year of life.[5] In a small subset of children, this coordinated progression of thumb function is impaired and congenital flexion deformities of the thumb are present. Congenital flexion deformities result from musculotendinous imbalance, joint abnormalities, and intrinsic tendon and tendon sheath anomalies. The most common causes of persistent congenital thumb flexion are congenital trigger thumb and congenital clasped thumb.

Supported in part by a Midcareer Investigator Award in Patient-Oriented Research (K24AR053120) from the National Institute of Arthritis and Musculoskeletal and Skin Diseases (Kevin C. Chung).
[a] Division of Plastic and Reconstructive Surgery, Department of Surgery, Stanford University Hospitals & Clinics, 770 Welch Road, Suite 400, Palo Alto, CA 94304, USA
[b] Section of Plastic Surgery, Department of Surgery, University of Michigan Medical School, 2130 Taubman Center, 1500 E. Medical Center Drive, Ann Arbor, MI 48109-0340, USA
* Corresponding author.
E-mail address: kecchung@umich.edu (K.C. Chung).

Hand Clin 25 (2009) 265–276
doi:10.1016/j.hcl.2008.12.008

CONGENITAL TRIGGER THUMB

Congenital trigger thumb is characterized by persistent flexion of the interphalangeal (IP) joint. The thumb is easily flexed; however, extension at the IP joint is impaired. True triggering is rare and motion at the metacarpophalangeal joint is unencumbered. The initial descriptions of triggering are attributed to Notta,[6] a French physician who described nodules occurring within the flexor tendons resulting in pathologic triggering of the affected digit. Notta's original reports were based on his experience with adult trigger finger; however, the term Notta's node has persisted only in descriptions of congenital trigger finger.

The age of onset, etiology, and treatment of congenital trigger thumb remain a matter of supposition and debate. Congenital trigger thumb is estimated to constitute 2.2% of all upper extremity congenital anomalies with an incidence of 1 in 2000 live births.[1,7] The diagnosis is typically made after 6 months of life. Attempts to establish the incidence at birth have provided substantial evidence that congenital trigger thumb is more likely acquired after birth and that the term "congenital trigger thumb" is in itself a misnomer. Rodgers and Waters[8] examined 1046 newborns, whereas Slakey and Hennrikus[9] examined 4719 newborns for the presence of thumb triggering at birth. No trigger thumbs were identified. Kikuchi and Ogino[10] examined 1166 neonates within 14 days of birth and found no congenital trigger thumbs. Of these 1166 patients, two patients went on to develop trigger thumbs within the first year of life. Authors have, however, pointed to cases of fraternal twins,[11] association with trisomy 13 (Pateau Syndrome)[12] and families with generational occurrence suggesting a heritable component or predisposition.[13]

Etiology

From a purely mechanical perspective, congenital trigger thumb results from a discrepancy between the flexor pollicis longus (FPL) tendon and the overlying flexor tendon sheath. Fusiform thickening of the FPL tendon, referred to as Notta's nodule, is pathognomonic of congenital trigger thumb. The nodule is characteristically palpable at the level of the metacarpophalangeal (MCP) joint. The strong flexors of the thumb allow the nodule to be pulled proximally, beneath the retinacular pulley system; however, the weaker extensor apparatus is unable to overcome the stenosis at the level of the first annular (A1) pulley. As a result the thumb takes on a persistent flexed position at the IP joint (**Fig. 1**).

The exact pathologic sequence resulting in congenital trigger thumb is not defined. Theories

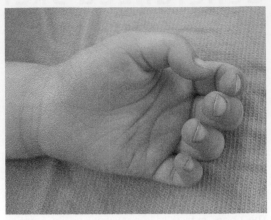

Fig. 1. A typical trigger thumb in a 5-year-old girl. Please note the flexion at the IP joint.

have focused on the two pathologic components: Notta's node and the A1 pulley. Microscopic examination of Notta's node reveals normal collagenous tendon architecture infiltrated with lymphocytes and monocytes, suggestive of traumatic inflammation.[14] This fusiform enlargement of the tendon resolves following surgical release of the A1 pulley.[15] The A1 pulley itself may be thickened and its anatomy variable. No studies have examined the anatomy of the digital pulley system in infants; however, numerous studies in the adult hand have demonstrated variable anatomy that may predispose the thumb to triggering. Schmidt and Fischer described[16] a Y-shaped fiber complex located at the base of the proximal phalanx in 90% of adult thumbs. They also described thin accessory pulley fibers located between the A1 pulley and this Y-shaped fiber complex, in effect, extending the A1 pulley complex. Bayat and colleagues[17] dissected 14 hands, describing a distinct annular pulley located between the A1 and the oblique pulley, which they designated the variable pulley. Variable anatomy exists within the fibrous pulley system that may contribute to the development of thumb triggering.

Histologic studies support the theory that tendon inflammation—manifest as enlargement of the FPL tendon—results in a discrepancy in size between the tendon and its associated pulley system. This discrepancy in size then contributes to further trauma and inflammation of the tendon and overlying retinacular pulley. What initiates this cycle of trauma and inflammation is a matter of supposition. Several authors speculate that the neonatal flexed thumb posture may produce chronic irritation of the FPL tendon with impingement occurring at the level of the A1 pulley, and that the stenosis may be exacerbated by the underlying cartilaginous sesamoids.[10,14] Other authors have proposed that anatomic aberrancy with congenital constriction at the A1 pulley may be the inciting event.[18]

Treatment

Not only does substantial debate exist regarding the etiology of congenital trigger finger but also regarding both the timing and appropriate treatment. Treatment options include: observation, splinting, range of motion exercises, and surgical release of the A1 pulley. Surgical intervention remains the mainstay of treatment. The A1 pulley may be approached through a transverse incision at the level of the MCP flexion crease, a Bruner-type incision crossing the flexion crease, or an axial incision placed proximal to the flexion crease. The radial and ulnar neurovascular bundles are carefully identified and retracted laterally as their course at this level is superficial. The proximal and distal extent of the A1 pulley is clearly identified and the pulley is divided with scissors or a number 15 scalpel. The oblique fibers of the retinacular pulley system are preserved. A Senn retractor is then placed deep to the FPL tendon and tendon excursion is tested to ensure adequate surgical release and unrestricted thumb motion. No resection or debulking of the FPL tendon is indicated because the Notta's node resolves once the A1 pulley has been released.[15] Recently, van Loveren and van der Bierzen[19] have questioned the classic teaching that A1 pulley release alone is necessary and sufficient to effectively release the congenital trigger thumb. They found that release of the A1 pulley alone was sufficient to cure this disease in only 19% of treated thumbs, whereas 13% were released with division of the variable pulley alone and 68% required release of both the A1 pulley and the variable pulley. The authors suggest that the identification of the region of stenosis and targeted release of this region alone is preferable to routine release of the A1 pulley. They report no increased incidence of bowstringing—even in cases where more extensive release was performed.

Surgical timing is likewise controversial. Dinham and Meggitt[20] note an increased risk of IP joint contracture in children undergoing surgical release after the age of 3 years. This assertion is refuted by several studies that demonstrate no residual contractures in children whose surgical treatment was delayed beyond the age of 3 years.[21–23]

Nonoperative treatments include observation, passive extension exercises, and splinting. Observation is based on the assumption that a spontaneous recovery rate exists. Dinham and Meggitt reviewed the natural history of congenital trigger thumb, citing a spontaneous resolution rate of 31% for children presenting before 6 months of age, 12% for those presenting between 6 and 12 months of age, and no spontaneous resolution in children presenting after the age of 1 year. Mulpruek and Prichasuk[24] reported a 24% spontaneous recovery rate. Tan and colleagues[21] have advocated passive extension exercises with or without extension splinting while the child is sleeping, reporting an overall success rate of 66% with nonoperative treatment. Resolution rates of 89% are noted for children younger than 1 year of age, decreasing to 50% in children treated after the age of 3 years.

Outcomes and Recommendation for Treatment

Spontaneous resolution of congenital trigger thumb occurs in up to 30% of patients, particularly those children diagnosed younger than 1 year of age, and this recovery may be facilitated by passive extension exercises and IP joint extension splinting. The vast majority of children with persistent IP joint contracture persisting beyond 1 year of age will require operation. The outcomes of operative intervention are universally reliable with a low incidence of complications; a 15-year follow-up in 21 patients demonstrates only minor deficits in IP joint extension in 23% on patients and no associated functional deficits. The most common complication was unsatisfactory scarring and contracture in one third of patients as a result of a longitudinal incision crossing the MP flexion crease. The authors emphasized the importance of a transverse incision to avoid scar contracture across the flexion surface.[25] Tan followed 72 patients treated with surgical release of the A1 pulley, noting a 1.4% recurrence rate and a 2.8% rate of wound infection. The recurrence occurred at 7 months and was attributed to inadequate release at the initial procedure.[21] Concern for bowstringing has been raised in cadaveric models in which the A1 and variable pulley are released;[17] however, van Loveren released the A1 and Av pulleys in 11 patients and reported no clinical evidence of bowstringing.[19]

The authors proceed with surgical release at one year of age. Waiting until this age has several advantages. First, in the majority of children, triggering will resolve spontaneously and will have done so. Second, the anatomic structures are of sufficient size to allow for facile identification and preservation of the neurovascular bundles as well as accurate division of the A1 pulley. Lastly, the risk of anesthesia is reduced. The authors prefer a Bruner type incision to allow for ample visualization and for the dissection to be carried distally should A1 pulley release alone not fully alleviate the stenosis. The authors routinely divide the A1 pulley. If triggering persists, the dissection is carried distally to identify and divide the residual region of stenosis, typically resulting from a variable pulley. The oblique pulley is preserved and the distal extent of the dissection is minimized in an effort to preserve the flexor sheath. The skin is closed with absorbable sutures and a soft dressing is applied.

CONGENITAL CLASPED THUMB

Congenital clasped thumb includes a spectrum of deformity in which the thumb is held in an adducted, flexed position within the palm. Although the condition is present at birth, the diagnosis is often delayed until after four months of life, when active extension of the thumb fails to develop. Several authors have referred to the clasped thumb deformity as a syndrome in itself; however, the condition is more accurately described as a physical finding that occurs in isolation or, more commonly, as a component of a syndrome, including arthrogryposis, wind-blown hand syndrome and a number of central nervous system disorders.[26–30]

Anatomy and Classification

In contrast to congenital trigger finger in which flexion occurs at the IP joint alone, congenital clasped thumb is characterized by adduction in combination with flexion at the MCP and IP joint. This posture results from an imbalance between the flexor and extensor mechanisms. Classification of the clasped thumb deformity was initially outlined by Weckesser and colleagues.[31] This classification scheme divides the deformity into four groups: Group I, characterized by weak or absent extensor tendons; Group II, characterized by weak of absent extensor tendons in association with flexion contractures of the other digits; Group III includes more complex deficiencies, joint abnormalities and thenar muscle hypoplasia; and Group IV includes all thumbs that are not easily classified into Groups I–III, including thumb duplication. This classification has proven cumbersome in the clinical context. McCarrol[32] proposed dividing the clasped thumb deformity into supple and complex types. The supple deformity is characterized by absence or hypoplasia of the extensor mechanism. The complex deformity includes MCP joint contracture, collateral ligament instability, thenar muscle absence or hypoplasia, and first web-space deficiency in addition to absence or hypoplasia of the extensor mechanism. Mih[33] proposed a modification of

McCarroll's classification in which: supple thumbs are classified as Type I; complex thumbs as Type II; and clasped thumbs in association with arthrogryposis and wind-blown hand as Type III. This classification is useful clinically with treatment varying in accordance with the classification.

Imbalance between the thumb flexor and extensor mechanisms is the principal feature of the congenital clasped thumb deformity. This imbalance is most often the result of hypoplasia or aplasia of the extensor pollicis brevis;[34–36] however, abnormalities of the extensor pollicis longus (EPL) and the abductor pollicis longus have been described.[37,38] The extensor pollicis brevis (EPB) inserts into the base of the proximal phalanx by stabilizing the MCP joint and allowing for extension at the level of the MCP joint as well as abduction of the thumb without rotation. The extensor pollicis longus inserts into the distal phalanx by providing extension at the IP joint, whereas the abductor pollicis longus inserts into the base of the thumb metacarpal, allowing for abduction at the level of the carpometacarpal (CMC) joint. Absence of the EPB results in flexion and instability at the MCP joint; absence of EPL results in flexion at the IP joint. Deficiency of the APL allows the thumb to be held in a tightly adducted position within the palm. Deficiency of the extensor components varies from complete absence of the tendons to thread-like hypoplasia, or discontinuity distal to the musculotendinous junction.[1,31]

Treatment

Reconstruction of the clasped thumb deformity requires an accurate assessment of the anatomic abnormalities and a combination of techniques specifically designed to reconstruct the deficient tissues and to reposition the thumb. Supple clasped thumbs are often amenable to splint therapy or reconstruction of the extensor mechanism alone; complex clasped thumbs require release of the MCP joint and first web-space adduction contractures as well as reconstruction of the thenar musculature and provision for additional tissue within the first web space.

The use of a short opponens splint has a central role in the treatment supple clasped thumb deformities. Splinting the thumb in a position of abduction and extension allows the extensor apparatus, which is typically hypoplastic, to develop and serves to weaken the thumb flexors and adductors. This therapy improves the balance between the thumb flexors and extensors. Splinting is initiated at 3–6 months of age. The splint is worn at all times for 3–6 months and night splinting alone is continued for up to one year. The majority of supple clasped thumb deformities will respond to splinting alone.

Surgical reconstruction is indicated in patients who have supple clasped thumb deformities that do not improve with splinting and in patients who have complex clasped thumb deformities. Supple clasped thumbs require reconstruction of the deficient extensor mechanism via tendon transfer (**Fig. 2**). A variety of tendon transfers have been described including the use of the extensor indicis proprius, brachioradialis, extensor carpi radialis longus, and flexor digitorum superficialis (FDS). The brachioradialis and the extensor carpi radialis longus tendons have limited functional excursion and require tendon lengthening or grafting to be useful as thumb extensors. The extensor indicis proprius is an ideal donor because this tendon is easily exposed within the fourth dorsal compartment just ulnar to the EDC to the index finger and its function is redundant. This tendon, however, is frequently absent in patients who have clasped thumb deformity.[32,33] FDS transfer for extensor reconstruction was first described by Crawford

and colleagues[39] in 1966. Presence of both FDS and flexor digitorum profundus to the long or middle finger is confirmed on pre-operative clinical examination. An oblique, Bruner type incision is made on the volar surface of the hand, overlying the proximal phalanx. The FDS is incised proximal to its insertion into the middle phalanx. The tendon is then passed proximally and retrieved via a longitudinal incision placed proximal to the carpal tunnel. The tendon is then rerouted through the first dorsal compartment via an incision place at the radial border of the wrist and is inserted into the proximal phalanx to reconstruct the EPB. The thumb is immobilized in a thumb spica or short opponens splint for 4 weeks.

Reconstruction of complex clasped thumb deformities requires not only reconstruction of the extensor mechanism but also release of the MCP and first web-space contracture, thenar muscle reconstruction, and soft tissue provision within the first web space. These soft tissue abnormalities are likely secondary to the congenitally flexed posture and may be relieved, to some degree,

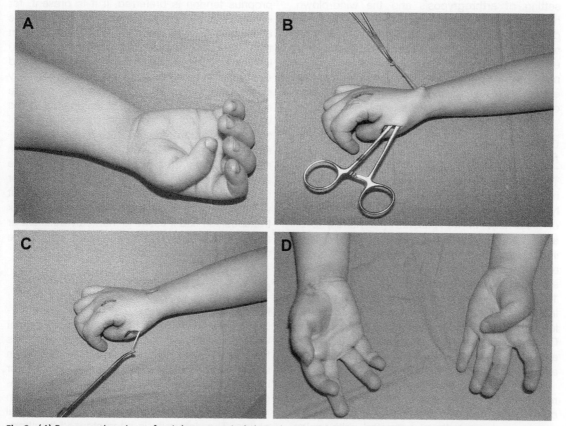

Fig. 2. (A) Preoperative view of a right congenital clasp thumb deformity in a 3-year-old boy. Patient did not have a functional EPL tendon, so an EIP tendon transfer was performed to extend the thumb. (B, C) Intraoperative views of the EIP tendon transfer. (D) 6-weeks postoperative picture. Note the improved extension of the reconstructed right thumb.

with preoperative splinting. Intraoperative evaluation and malleable decision-making are necessary to achieve a good functional result without undue surgical manipulation of the thumb. Release of the MCP flexion contracture requires division of the volar plate and flexor pollicis longus lengthening, which is accomplished with a stair-step lengthening incision in the FPL tendon. Lengthening is performed at the level of the wrist to avoid scarring and adhesion within zones II and III. Correction of the MCP flexion contracture may result in laxity of the ulnar collateral ligament, requiring imbrications to stabilize the MCP joint. The thenar musculature is examined intraoperatively and any deficiency requires reconstruction with an opponensplasty. Either the FDS or the abductor digiti minimi may be used. Provision for soft tissue within the first web space is provided with a full thickness skin graft, four-flap Z-plasty, or with an index transposition flap.[40] The adductor pollicis and first dorsal interosseous are examined through this exposure and myotomies performed if the web space remains tight despite soft tissue rearrangement.

Complex clasped thumbs occurring in the setting of arthrogryposis and the wind-blown hand deformity present an additional level of complexity. In these cases, donor tendons, such as the FDS, extensor indicis proprius (EIP) and wrist extensors, may be absent. Thenar muscle hypoplasia is often particularly pronounced and consideration should be given to extra-epiphyseal fusion of the MCP joint to provide for a stable thumb.

Outcomes and Recommendations for Treatment

The outcomes of congenital clasped thumb treatment vary proportionally with the degree of underlying deformity. Tsuyuguchi examined the results of treatment in 43 patients (75 hands) over a 10-year period. These patients were subdivided into groups corresponding to supple, complex, and clasped thumbs associated with arthrogryposis; 42 hands were treated with splinting alone and 16 hands underwent operative treatment. Surgical indications were: MP extension or CMC abduction less than 30° and failure of splint therapy. Outcomes were rated as excellent, good, fair, and poor based on extension at the MCP joint and abduction at the CMC joint.

Splint therapy uniformly provided excellent results in 19 of 19 patients treated with supple clasped thumbs. On the other hand, 9 of 12 complex clasped thumbs treated with splint therapy were rated as excellent and 3 of 12 were rated as fair. Clasped thumbs in the setting of arthrogryposis generally responded poorly to splint

therapy with 3 of 11 rated as excellent, 2 of 11 as good, 5 of 11 as fair and one as poor. The average duration of splinting varied from 3.2 months for supple clasped thumbs to 7 months for clasped thumbs in the setting of arthrogryposis. Surgical results varied inversely with the severity of the preoperative deformity. Of the eight complex clasped thumbs treated surgically, five results were rated as excellent, two good, and one fair. Of the eight clasped thumbs associated with arthrogryposis, four results were rated as excellent, one good, two fair, and one poor (**Table 1**).[41]

The authors routinely perform splinting for both supple and complex clasped thumb deformities. In agreement with Tsuyuguchi's results, the authors have found few supple clasped thumbs that have not responded appropriately to splint therapy alone. Splinting of complex clasped thumbs reduces the first web contracture and may minimize MCP joint contracture. The authors consider surgical intervention at the age of 12–15 months in patients who have not responded to splint therapy and in whom CMC abduction and MP extension are limited. Use the extensor indicis proprius tendon is preferred, if it is present, for extensor tendon reconstruction. In the absence of the EIP, the authors prefer FDS transfer from the long finger over using the extensor carpi radialis longus or the brachioradialis given their limited excursion. In their practices, the authors routinely explore the MCP joint and release the volar plate if this joint is tight. The FPL is lengthened at the wrist to avoid adhesions within zones II and III of the flexor tendon sheath. They prefer to reconstruct the deficient thenar musculature with an abductor digiti minimi oppenensplasty. The authors perform partial release of the adductor pollicis and first dorsal interosseous. Deficient web-space soft tissue is provided with an index transposition flap if tissue is markedly deficient or a four-flap Z-plasty if only moderate soft tissue deficiency exists.

MADELUNG DEFORMITY

Madelung's deformity is a rare disorder characterized by shortening of the forearm with a bayonet wrist deformity. Madelung's deformity accounts for only 1.7% of all congenital hand anomalies and its etiology remains uncertain.[1] Congenital or idiopathic Madelung deformity should be distinguished from pseudo-Madelung deformity, which results form trauma or infection of the radial physis. The deformity is characterized by shortening and curvature of the radius, a widened distal radioulnar joint, dorsal luxation of the distal ulna, and a triangular arrangement of the carpal bones

Table 1
Congenital clasped thumb

Type	Description	Anatomic Abnormalities	Treatment
Type I	Supple clasped thumb	Hypoplastic extensor tendon(s): EPB, EPL, APB; Absent extensor tendon(s): EPB, EPL, APB	Opponens splint; tendon transfer: EIP, FDS, ECR or brachioradialis
Type II	Complex clasped thumb	Hypoplastic/absent extensor tendon(s); MCP joint contracture; adduction/first web-space contracture; Thenar muscle hypoplasia	Opponens splint; tendon transfer; Volar plate release; FPL-lengthening myotomy: adductor pollicis, first dorsal interosseous; skin graft; 4-flap Z-plasty; index transposition flap; opponensplasty: ADM, FDS
Type III	Clasped thumb associated with arthrogryposis and wind-blown hand	Same as complex clasped thumb with arthrogryposis of the upper extremity	Same as complex clasped thumb

Abbreviations: ADM, abductor digiti minimi; APB, abductor pollicis brevis; ECR, extensor carpi radialis.

that result in proximo-volar subluxation of the carpus and a step-off or bayonet deformity.[42,43] The ulnar and dorsal curvature of the distal radius results from deficient growth of the volar and ulnar aspect of the distal radius physis (**Fig. 3**).

Etiology

Anatomic changes are not readily apparent until childhood or early adolescence; however, associations with achondroplasia, Turner's syndrome, and Leri-Weill syndrome provide evidence for a congenital etiology.[44] Several authors have

proposed that Madelung's deformity represents one end of the spectrum of dyschondrosteosis, rather than an isolated anomaly.[45,46] Zebela and Manske examined 18 patients (31 extremities) with Madelung deformity. Patients were categorized as having involvement of the entire radius, and 10 of the patients demonstrated involvement of the distal radius alone. They found that average patient height for patients with distal radius involvement was in the 24th percentile, whereas the height of patients with involvement of the entire radius was in the 9th percentile. Average radial lengths were significantly shorter than

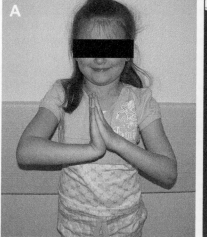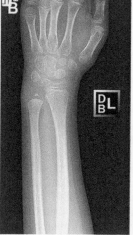

Fig. 3. (*A*) Photograph of a 6-year-old girl with progressive deformity of the wrist, demonstrating a typical Madelung's appearance. (*B*) Radiograph showing a dorsal-riding distal ulna and collapse of the ulnar column of the distal radius epiphyseal plate.

age-matched controls in both groups.[46] These findings strongly support the theory that Madelung deformity has a strong genetic component and falls along the spectrum of dyschondrosteosis.

Deficient longitudinal growth along the ulnar and volar aspect of the radius physis explains the characteristic pronounced radial inclination and volar tilt of the distal radius; however, the etiology of this asymmetric physeal growth remains a matter of supposition. Etiologic theories have included focal vascular insufficiency to the ulnar physis as well as mechanical constraints resulting from the tethering of the lunate to the distal radius.[47,48] Greater controversy exists regarding the clinical and operative treatment of patients who have Madelung deformity.

Treatment

Patients who have Madelung deformity exhibit restricted range of motion, particularly in extension of the wrist and supination at the distal radioulnar joint. Vickers and Neilsen[48] report an average loss of supination of 31° in 24 wrists. Schmidt-Rohlfing and colleagues[44] reported a full range of motion in 36% of patients, restricted motion in all directions in 19% of patients, and deficiency in at least on direction in 45% of patients, noting that the majority of these patients exhibited limitation of supination. Pain is a common complaint, particularly in adolescence; however, this pain is often transient and may be improved with orthotic splints.[49] Salon reported daily pain resulting in functional impairment in 50% of patients who have Madelung deformity.[50] Schmidt-Rohlfing[44] reported pain in 77% of patients; however, only 16% of patients experienced pain at rest and with daily life activities. The goals of operative treatment are primarily relief of pain, correction of the cosmetic wrist deformity, and preservation or improvement in range of motion through the application of corrective osteotomies, physiolysis, ulnar shortening and ligamentous release.

Correction of the Madelung deformity in patients at skeletal maturity requires restoration of the distal radius anatomy. Corrective osteotomies of the radius are designed to restore a physiologic distal radial inclination of 22°. This correction may be performed via opening wedge osteotomies on the ulnar aspect of the radius or closing wedge osteotomies on the radial aspect. A volar osteotomy may be performed in an effort to restore a normal volar tilt of 11°. Osteotomies are performed at the level of the metaphysis. Ulnar resection is performed to restore neutral ulnar variance, allowing for reduction of the distal radioulnar joint.

Over the past 20 years, operative intervention that seeks to prevent the development of severe Madelung deformity has evolved. Vickers[48,51,52] describes an abnormality in the distal radial physis as well as an abnormal volar ligament tethering the distal radius and the lunate. This ligamentous tether fixes the lunate in a proximal position, resisting longitudinal growth and thinning the epiphysis via compression. Physiolysis and release of this taut volar ligament before physeal fusion allow for compensatory growth at the volar aspect of the distal radius. Physiolysis is performed via a volar transverse incision placed proximal to the most proximal wrist crease. Dissection is carried down to the pronator quadratus, protecting the median nerve and radial artery. The pronator quadratus is released. The ligamentous tether between the lunate and the distal radius is released. A sagittal osteotomy of the distal radius is performed to isolate the ulnar aspect of the physis, and a fat graft is placed in contact with the physis to fill the sagittal osteotomy defect. A volar splint is applied for 2–4 weeks.

Outcomes and Recommendations for Treatment

The outcomes of surgical treatment of Madelung's deformity are difficult to compare because of the broad spectrum of presentation, as well as the variable operative indications and timing of operation used by hand surgeons. The operation rate is highly variable among published series. Salon reported on 14 wrists, 11 of which were treated operatively for daily pain and functional impairment in everyday activities.[50] In contrast, Schmidt-Rohlfing and colleagues[44] reported on a series of 31 patients in which five patients underwent operative treatment for persistent pain. Vickers and Neilsen[48] reported a series of 17 patients in which seven patients underwent operative treatment. All authors have reported adequate restoration of radial inclination and volar tilt, as well as acceptable pain relief. Only Vickers[48] reports an increase in wrist range of motion, citing an improvement in supination by an average of 23°.

The authors of this article have found that the majority of patients adapt well to the deformity with a functional range of motion and only intermittent wrist pain. The authors do not routinely perform prophylactic physiolyis or release Vicker's ligament; rather, they prefer to operate only when pain is persistent or deformity so severe that it impairs wrist function in activities of daily living.

ACHONDROPLASIA

Achondroplasia is a characteristic skeletal disorder resulting from deficient endochondral ossification manifest as longitudinal growth retardation. The incidence of achondroplasia is between 0.5 and 1.5 in 10,000 live births. The disorder is inherited in an autosomal dominant fashion with complete penetrance, and 80% of cases are the result of de novo mutations. The disease is caused by mutation of the Fibroblast Growth Factor Receptor 3 (FGFR3) gene on the short arm of chromosome 4.[53] The FGFR3 gene encodes a tyrosine kinase trans-membrane receptor that, when bound with its ligand, inhibits physeal growth. The mutated receptor is constitutively activated, requiring no ligand binding for activation.

The physes of patients who have achondroplasia demonstrate a histologically normal progression of columnization, hypertrophy, degeneration, calcification and ossification; however, the growth is quantitatively reduced resulting in longitudinal deficiency.[54] Subperiosteal membranous ossification is unaffected and, consequently, the bones exhibit normal diameter. These characteristic changes are found in all the long bones and are particularly pronounced in the humerus and femur, leading to rhizomelic phocomelia in which the extremities are disproportionately short in the proximal segment.

Retarded longitudinal growth is apparent in the hand and forearm, leading to characteristic deformities including the trident hand deformity, variable finger length, and restricted elbow extension. The trident hand deformity is a cardinal finding in patients who have achondroplasia and is characterized by divergence of the phalanges. The deformity most commonly involves the long and ring finger and is the result of asymmetric growth at the level of the proximal phalanx.[55] Both in utero and until adolescence, growth at the ulnar aspect of the proximal phalangeal physis of the long finger, and at the radial aspect of the ring finger is dominant. This asymmetry of growth leads to divergence of the long and ring fingers manifest as a trident deformity, most noticeable when the fingers are in full extension. Throughout adolescence, the asymmetric growth is corrected and, by adulthood, the deformity typically resolves. Asymmetric longitudinal growth of the fingers is also characteristic. The most common presentation is deficient length of the long finger, making this finger comparable in length to the ring finger. This discrepancy is of little functional consequence.

Although patients who have achondroplasia often exhibit generalized joint hypermobility, restricted motion is characteristic at the elbow and distal radioulnar joint. Bailey[55] examined the hand and forearms of 41 patients who have achondroplasia, documenting limited extension in 93% and restricted supination in 33%. This limitation in motion was typically bilateral but rarely symmetric. He also noted that these restrictions tended to increase with age. Anatomic studies reveal no single cause; however, many deformities include anomalies of the radial head, subluxation or the radial head, humeral impingement of the olecranon tip within the olecranon fossa, incongruity of the olecranon fossa, and tight capsules, ligaments and tendons about the elbow joint.

Achondroplasia is characterized by a host of upper extremity anomalies; however, these deformities are rarely so severe as to require operative treatment. Ilizarov distraction osteogenesis has been employed to lengthen the humerus and femur. No reports of the application of this technique to the forearm and hand have been published in the existing literature, underscoring the fact that these deformities are rarely of substantive functional consequence to warrant intervention.

MARFAN SYNDROME AND CONGENITAL CONTRACTURAL ARACHNODACTYLY

Although achondroplasia is marked by a deficiency of longitudinal growth, Marfan syndrome is notable for excessive longitudinal growth creating thin, spider-like fingers. Marfan syndrome is an autosomal dominant disorder with variable expressivity that is now known to be caused by a host of mutations of the Fibrillin 1 (FBN1) gene located on the long arm of chromosome 15.[56,57] Marfan syndrome occurs in two to three per 10,000 live births and with 70% to 75% of affecting individuals born to an affected parent.[53] Molecular defects in the Fibrillin 1 gene are responsible for impaired structural integrity of the skeletal, ocular, and cardiovascular systems.

Fibrillin is an integral component of the extracellular matrix and is specifically localized within microfibrils, which form a scaffold for elastin deposition.[58] The mechanism by which mutation of Fibrillin 1 results in a myriad of systemic anomalies spanning multiple organ systems remains a mystery. Initial theories focused on the role of Fibrillin within the structure of the microfibrils. Changes within the fibrillin molecule would result in disruption of the microfibrils, altering elastin deposition, and consequently, disrupting the ordered architecture of the extracellular matrix.[59] This theory, however, does not provide a plausible mechanism for some of the most salient features of the Marfan phenotype including long bone and rib overgrowth, as well as alterations of muscle growth and fat metabolism. Recent theories have focused on the interaction between Fibrillin 1 and Transforming Growth Factor β (TGF-β), a ubiquitous mediator of inflammation. Fibrillin may bind and sequester TGB-β, preventing inflammation that weakens the extracellular matrix and connective tissue.[60] Despite these advances, a complete understanding of the pathophysiology of Marfan syndrome remains elusive.

Arachnodactyly is one of the most prominent clinical features and constitutes a major criterion for the diagnosis of Marfan syndrome. Patients who have arachnodactyly exhibit long, thin, often hyperextensible fingers. Positive wrist and thumb signs are characteristic of the diagnosis. The wrist test (Walker-Murdoch) is performed by having patients wrap their fingers around the contralateral wrists. If the distal phalanges of the thumb and small finger overlap, the test is considered positive. The thumb test is performed by having the patient clasp their thumb within the palm. If the thumb projects beyond the ulnar border of the hand, the test is considered positive.[53]

Congenital contractural arachnodactyly (Beals syndrome) is an autosomal dominant disorder that is closely related and frequently confused with Marfan syndrome. The disease is characterized by a marfanoid habitus, arachnodactyly, camptodactyly, clasped thumbs, crumpled ears, and mild contractures of the elbows, knees and hips. Patients often exhibit scoliosis and mitral valve prolapse, and a small subset develop aortic root dilation. Beals syndrome results from mutations within the Fibrillin2 (FBN2) in contrast to the FBN1 gene implicated in Marfan syndrome.[61] Akin to Marfan syndrome, arachnodactyly is present; however, congenital contracture of the proximal interphalangeal joints is marked and distinguishes the characteristic hand findings in congenital contractural arachnodactyly. This contracture improves with time and no operative therapy is indicated.[62]

SUMMARY

Congenital skeletal abnormalities encompass a broad range of disorders including congenital flexion deformities of the thumb, Madelung deformity, and general skeletal and connective tissue disorders. Disorders may be isolated to the hand and forearm or they may be reflective of a systemic disease process, as in the cases of achondroplasia and Marfan syndrome.

Congenital flexion deformities of the thumb result in significant functional limitations. Most commonly, this deformity is the result of a congenital trigger finger or a congenital clasped thumb. Both disorders are often delayed in diagnosis by the natural flexed posture of the newborn's thumb. Congenital trigger finger results from a discrepancy between the flexor tendon and the retinacular tendon sheath allowing full flexion but limiting extension at the interphalangeal joint. Many patients will respond to splinting alone; however, surgical release of the A1 pulley is reliable and associated minimal morbidity. In contrast, congenital clasped thumb results from an imbalance between the thumb flexors and extensors and it is more commonly associated with neurologic and syndromic disorders. Supple clasped thumbs respond reliably to splinting alone; however, complex clasped thumbs require reconstruction of the extensor mechanism, release of intrinsic MCP joint and adduction contracture, and provision for soft tissue within the first web space. This complex reconstruction underscores the importance of accurate identification of the underlying anatomic abnormality and meticulous, targeted correction of each abnormal component.

Madelung deformity of the wrist results from abnormal growth at the ulnar and volar aspect of the physis contributing to a bayonet wrist deformity. Functional limitations are often modest; persistent pain occurs in a subset of patients. Operative treatments are reserved for patients who have persistent pain and severe, functionally limiting deformities of the wrist. Operative indications, choice of operative technique, and the timing of operative intervention remain controversial.

ACKNOWLEDGMENTS

The authors acknowledge Allison Pushman for her organization and coordination of this article.

REFERENCES

1. Flatt AE. The care of congenital hand anomalies. St. Louis (MO): CV Mosby; 1977.
2. McCarroll HR. Congenital anomalies: a 25-year overview. J Hand Surg [Am] 2000;25(6):1007–37.
3. Frantz CH, O'Rahilly R. Congenital skeletal limb deficiencies. J Bone Joint Surg [Am] 1961;43:1202–24.
4. Swanson AB. A classification for congenital limb malformations. J Hand Surg [Am] 1976;1A:8–22.
5. Gessell A. An atlas of infant behaviour. New Haven (CT): Yale University Press; 1934. p. 243–9.
6. Notta A. Recherches sur une affection particuliere des gaines tendineuses de la main, caracterisee par le development d'une nodosite sur le trajet des tendons flechisseurs des doigts et par

l'empechement de leurs mouvements. Arch Gen Med 1850;24:142–61 [in French].

7. Ger E, Kupcha P, Ger D. The management of trigger thumb in children. J Hand Surg [Am] 1991;16A:944–7.

8. Rodgers WB, Waters PW. Incidence of trigger digits in newborns. J Hand Surg [Am] 1994;19A:364–8.

9. Slakey JB, Hennrikus WL. Acquired thumb flexion contrature in children: congenital trigger thumb. J Bone Joint Surg [Br] 1996;78B:481–3.

10. Kikuchi N, Ogino T. Incidence and development of trigger thumb in children. J Hand Surg [Am] 2006; 31A:541–3.

11. Bollinger JA, Fahey JJ. Snapping thumb in infants and children. J Pediatr 1952;41:445–50.

12. Dobyns JH. Trigger digits. In: Green DP, editor. Operative hand surgery. 2nd edition. New York: Churchill Livingstone; 1988. p. 374–8.

13. Shim VC, Admire AA, Heidenreich RA, et al. Autosomal dominant inheritance pattern for trigger thumb. Plast Reconstr Surg 2002;109:240–1.

14. Spreecher EE. Trigger thumb in infants. J Bone Joint Surg 1949;31A:672–4.

15. van den Borne MPJ, Custers FP, van der Aa JPW, et al. Knappende dium bij 38 Kindren: Goede Resultaten Van Operatie op Korte en Lange Termijn. NTVG 2000;144:374–7 [in Dutch].

16. Schmidt HM, Fischer G. Die Verstarkungsbander der Sehnenscheide des M. Flexor Pollicis Longus. Handchir Mikrochir Plast Chir 1999;31:362–6 [in German].

17. Bayat A, Shaaban H, Giakas G, et al. The pulley system of the thumb: anatomic and biomechanical study. J Hand Surg [Am] 2002;27A:628–35.

18. Hueston JT, Wilson WF. The aetiology of trigger thumb. Hand 1972;4:257–60.

19. van Loveren M, van der Biezen JJ. The congenital trigger thumb: is release of the first annular pulley alone sufficient to resolve the triggering? Ann Plast Surg 2007;58:335–7.

20. Dinham JM, Meggitt BF. Trigger thumbs in children. a review of the natural history and indications for treatment in 105 patients. J Bone Joint Surg [Br] 1952;56B:153–5.

21. Tan AHC, Lam KS, Lee EH. The treatment outcome of trigger thumb in children. J Pediatr Orthop 2002;11:256–9.

22. Dunsmuir RA, Sherlock DA. The outcome of treatment of trigger thumb in children. J bone Joint Surg [Br] 2000;82:736–8.

23. Skov O, Bach A, Hammer A. Trigger thumbs in children: a follow-up study of 37 children below 15 years of age. J Hand Surg [Br] 1990;15B:466–7.

24. Malpruek P, Prichasuk S. Spontaneous recovery of trigger thumbs in children. J Hand Surg [Br] 1998; 23B:255–7.

25. McAdams TR, Blevins FT, Martin TP, et al. Long-term follow-up of surgical release of the a(1) pulley in childhood trigger thumb. J Pediatr Orthop 2002;22:41–3.

26. Dangles CJ, Bilos ZJ. Surgical correction of thumb deformity in arthrogryposis multiplex congenita. Hand 1981;13:55–8.

27. Fransen E, Lemmon V, Van Camp G, et al. CRASH syndrome: clinical spectrum of corpus callosum hypoplasia, retardation, adducted thumbs, spastic paresis, and hydrocephalus due to mutations in one single gene, L1. Eur J Hum Genet 1995;3: 273–84.

28. Legius E, Kaepernick L, Higgins JV, et al. Fine mapping of X-linked clasped thumb and mental retardation (MASA syndrome) in Xq28. Clin Genet 1994;45:165–8.

29. Mochizuki Y, Suyehiro Y, Ihara Y, et al. Congenital hydrocephalus and clasped thumbs: two cases of brothers in a family. Brain Dev 1981;3:407–9.

30. Straussberg R, Blatt I, Brand N, et al. X-linked mental retardation with bilateral clasped thumbs: report of another affected family. Clin Genet 1991; 40:337–42.

31. Weckesser EC, Reed JR, Heiple KG. Congenital clasped thumb (congenital flexion-adduction deformity of the thumb). A syndrome, not a specific entity. J Bone Joint Surg [Am] 1968;50A:1417–28.

32. McCarrol HR. Congenital flexion deformities of the thumb. Hand Clin 1985;1:567–75.

33. Mih AD. Congenital clasped thumb. Hand Clin 1998; 1:77–84.

34. Broadbent TR, Woolf RM. Flexion-adduction deformity of the thumb-congenital clasped thumb. Plast Reconstr Surg 1964;34:612–6.

35. Gold AM, Perlman RD. Congenital clasped thumb deformity, case report. Bull Hosp Joint Dis 1968; 29:255–8.

36. White JW, Jensen WE. The infant's persistent thumb-clutched hand. J Bone Joint Surg [Am] 1952;34A: 680–8.

37. Zadek I. Congenital absence of the extensor pollicis longus of both thumbs. Operation and cure. J Bone Joint Surg [Br] 1934;16B:432–4.

38. Miller JW. Pollex varus: a report of two cases. Univ Hosp Bull Ann Arbor 1943;10:10–1.

39. Crawford HH, Horton CE, Adamson JE. Congenital aplasia or hypoplasia of the thumb and finger extensor tendons. J Bone Joint Surg [Am] 1966;48: 82–91.

40. Spinner M. Fashioned transposition flap for soft tissue adduction contracture of the thumb. Plast Reconstr Surg 1969;44:345–8.

41. Tsuyuguchi Y, Masada K, Kawabata H, et al. Congenital clasped thumb: a review of 43 cases. J Hand Surg [Am] 1985;10:613–8.

42. Madelung O. Die spontane subluxation der hand nach vorne, verh. Dtsch gese Chir 1878;7:259–76 [in German].

43. Arora AS, Chung KC. Otto W. Madelung and the recognition of Madelung's deformity. J Hand Surg [Am] 2006;31A:177–82.

44. Schmidt-Rohlfing B, Schwobel B, Pauschert R, et al. Madelung deformity: clinical features, therapy and results. J Pediatr Orthop 2001;10:344–8.

45. Herdman RC, Langer LO, Good RA. Dyschondrosteosis: the most common cause of Madelung's deformity. J Pediatr 1966;68:432–41.

46. Zebala LP, Manske PR, Goldfarb CA. Madelung's deformity: a spectrum of presentation. J Hand Surg [Am] 2007;32A:1393–401.

47. Nielson JB. Madelung's deformity. A follow-up study of 26 cases and a review of the literature. Acta Orthop Scand 1977;48:379–84.

48. Vickers D, Neilsen G. Madelung deformity: surgical prophylaxis (physiolysis) during the late growth period by resection of the dyschondrosteosis lesion. J Hand Surg [Br] 1992;17B:401–7.

49. Lamb D. Madeulung deformity. J Hand Surg [Br] 1988;13B:3–4.

50. Salon A, Serra M, Pouliquen JC. Long-term follow-up of surgical correction of Madelung's deformity with conservation of the distal radioulnar joint in teenagers. J Hand Surg [Br] 2000;25B:22–5.

51. Vickers DW. Premature incomplete fusion of the growth plate: causes and treatment by resection (physiolysis) in 15 cases. Aust N Z J Surg 1980;50:393–401.

52. Vickers DW. Langenskiold's operation for congenital malformation of bone producing Madelung's deformity and clinodactyly. [abstract]. J Bone Joint Surg [Br] 1984;66:778.

53. Chen H. Atlas of genetic diagnosis and counseling. New Jersey: Humana Press; 2006. p. 15–22, 619–29.

54. Horton WA, Hood OJ, Machado MA, et al. Growth plate cartilage studies in achondroplasia. Basic Life Sci 1988;48:81–9.

55. Bailey JA. Elbow and other upper limb deformities in achondroplasia. Clin Orthop Relat Res 1971;80:75–8.

56. Dietz HC, Cutting GR, Pyeritz RE, et al. Marfan syndrome caused by a recurrent De Novo missense mutation in the fibrillin gene. Nature 1991;352:337–9.

57. Robinson PN, Godfrey M. The molecular genetics of Marfan syndrome and related microfibrillopathies. J Med Genet 2000;37:9–25.

58. Byers PH. Determination of the molecular basis of Marfan syndrome: a growth industry. J Clin Invest 2004;114:161–3.

59. Eldadah ZA, Brenn T, Furthmayer H, et al. Expression of a mutant human fibrillin allele upon a normal human or murine genetic background recapitulates a Marfan cellular phenotype. J Clin Invest 1995;95:874–80.

60. Pyeritz RE. A small molecule for a large disease. N Engl J Med 2008;358:2829–31.

61. Lee B, Godfrey M, Vitale E, et al. Linkage of Marfan syndrome and a phenotypically related disorder to two different fibrillin genes. Nature 1991;352:330–4.

62. Viljoen D. Congenital contractural arachnodactyly (Beals syndrome). J Med Genet 1994;31:640–3.

Congenital Differences About the Elbow

Scott H. Kozin, MD[a,b,*]

KEYWORDS

- Congenital • Elbow • Synostosis • Arthrogryposis
- Pterygium • Multiple hereditary exostosis

Certain congenital differences immediately impair elbow motion and function, whereas other ailments slowly limit elbow motion or cause instability. Diagnoses that immediately impair elbow function are: synostosis (including proximal radio-ulnar, radiohumeral, ulnohumeral), arthrogryposis, and pterygium. Congenital differences that affect elbow motion or stability over time include: multiple hereditary exostosis, Ollier disease, osteogenesis imperfecta, skeletal dysplasia, nail patella syndrome, and Gorham disease. In either case, the child's ability to perform activities of daily living and to participate in recreation is diminished. The impairment is related to the deficit in elbow or forearm motion, the overall length of the limb, the degree of ipsilateral hand function, and the status of the contralateral limb. This article discusses congenital differences that affect the elbow, with an emphasis on diagnosis and treatment. In some cases, surgery is effective in enhancing function. In other cases, observation is preferable because children possess remarkable ability to adapt without surgery.

CONGENITAL DIFFERENCES THAT DIRECTLY IMPAIR ELBOW FUNCTION
Synostosis

Synostosis is a generic term that indicates an osseous union between bones that are normally separated.[1–3] Clinically, however, there is a spectrum of presentation that varies with the degree of joint development and the amount of synostosis. In other words, the motion can range from full, unrestricted movement to no motion in cases when the bones are fused. The variability of motion is most notable about the forearm joint. Many children present to the office with limited pronation or supination. Mild deficits often are unrecognized until the child is older when the necessary activities of daily living become more complicated (eg, toileting, self-feeding). A history of trauma may or may not be present. Radiographs may be normal or demonstrate subtle findings about the radiocapitellar and proximal radioulnar joints (**Fig. 1**). An understanding of the continuum from normal anatomy to rigid synostosis prevents an unnecessary work-up and unsuccessful surgery.

Synostosis across the elbow can be in a longitudinal direction (ie, ulnar–humeral or radial–humeral) or in a transverse path across the proximal radioulnar joint.[1,2] Radiohumeral synostosis most commonly occurs in ulnar deficiency, but can be part of a synostosis syndrome, such as Herrmann multiple synostosis syndrome.[1,4] Proximal radioulnar joint synostosis can occur in isolation or can be found in a variety of syndromes, including trisomy (13 or 21) and fetal alcohol syndrome.[1]

Radiohumeral synostosis

Radiohumeral or ulnohumeral synostosis impairs elbow flexion and extension. The functional impact depends upon the elbow position, hand function, compensatory surrounding joint motion, and status of contralateral limb. Because radiohumeral synostosis most commonly occurs in children with ulnar deficiency (type IV), bilateral involvement and hand impairment are prevalent.[1] The child with ulnar deficiency is often born with the hand against

a Department of Orthopaedic Surgery, Temple University, Philadelphia, PA, USA
b Upper Extremity Center of Excellence, Shriners Hospitals for Children, 3551 North Broad Street, Philadelphia, PA 19140, USA
* Shriners Hospitals for Children, 3551 North Broad Street, Philadelphia, PA 19140.
E-mail address: skozin@shrinenet.org

Hand Clin 25 (2009) 277–291
doi:10.1016/j.hcl.2008.12.007

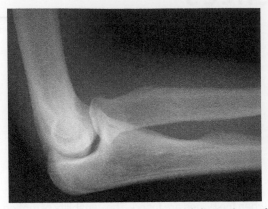

Fig. 1. A 14-year-old child presents with limited arc of forearm rotation (active pronation 45° and active supination 40°). Lateral radiograph reveals abnormal development of radiocapitellar joint with enlarged flattened radial head. (*Courtesy of* Shriners Hospital for Children, Philadelphia, PA; with permission.)

the flank, which positions the hand facing backward (**Fig. 2**). Treatment recommendations have varied from observation to corrective osteotomy to reposition the limb into a more functional location. In the past, I have improved limb position by way of osteotomy through the fusion mass. This can be accomplished acutely at the time of surgery or slowly with distraction osteogenesis. I have noticed, however, that children born with their hands facing backward often achieved similar positioning as those children who underwent surgery. In addition, their functional limitations were further lessened by their amazing compensatory motion (**Fig. 3**). The ability to compensate is unclear, but may be related to excessive surrounding joint motion or forces across the growth plate changing bony torsion. Nonetheless, the results are impressive and I now reserve osteotomy for recalcitrant cases that present with persistent poor limb position despite growth and development.

The limb with radiohumeral synostosis is often short owing to lack of growth plates. Limb lengthening has been recommended to improve workable reach space. However, distraction lengthening must be approached with great caution because the complication rate is high and the preoperative goals often unobtainable. Furthermore, limb lengthening can move the hand further from the face and adversely impact function. Therefore, considerable thought and evaluation are necessary before limb lengthening. An occupational therapy evaluation is invaluable to include an assessment of preoperative goals to prevent disappointment to both the patient and the surgeon.

Proximal radioulnar joint synostosis

Proximal radioulnar joint (PRUJ) synostosis is bilateral about 50% of the time and may be inheritable (**Fig. 4**).[2,3,5,6] Forearm motion must be assessed at the radial styloid and ulnar head (distal radioulnar joint) to avoid measuring wrist motion instead of forearm movement (**Fig. 5**). Anteroposterior and lateral elbow radiographs are necessary because the synostosis is nearly always about the PRUJ (**Fig. 6**). In the young child, the connection is initially cartilaginous but eventually ossifies to a bony connection. A concomitant radial head dislocation may be present. Advanced imaging studies are not necessary.

Shoulder and wrist motion is able to compensate for a lack of forearm rotation during many activities of early childhood. Shoulder abduction compensates for deficient pronation and shoulder adduction compensates for deficient supination (**Fig. 7**). Additionally, children with deficient forearm rotation will develop excessive wrist intercarpal rotation.[5] Therefore, a delay in presentation is common until the complexities of daily activities amplify, such as catching a ball, self-feeding, or toileting (**Fig. 8**). Common complaints from a pronation deficit are difficulties with keyboarding and tabletop activities. Common difficulties from a supination deficiency are eating, washing one's face, catching a ball, and using a soap dispenser. Many children present after unrelated trivial trauma, which alerts the parents to the absent forearm rotation.

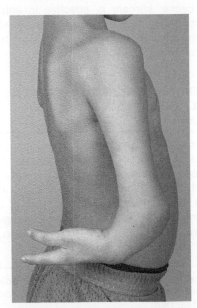

Fig. 2. A 4-year-old child with bilateral ulnar deficiencies and right hand facing backward. (*Courtesy of* Shriners Hospital for Children, Philadelphia, PA; with permission.)

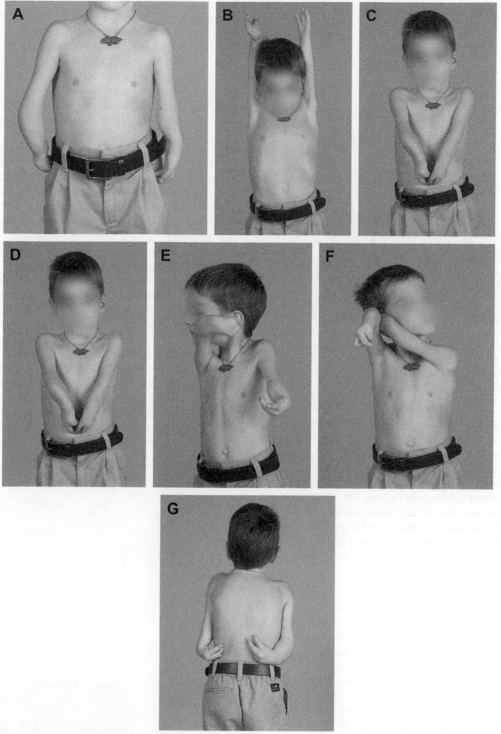

Fig. 3. A 6-year-old child with untreated bilateral ulnar deficiency. (*A*) Resting posture with left hand facing backward. (*B*) Overhead reach. (*C*) Midline activity. (*D*) Touching top of head for washing hair. (*E*) Touching left ear with right hand. (*F*) Touching left ear with right hand using left arm as assist. (*G*) Reaching back with both hands. (*Courtesy of* Shriners Hospital for Children, Philadelphia, PA; with permission.)

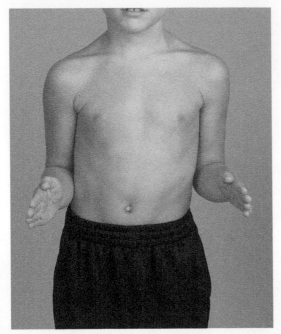

Fig. 4. A 7-year-old child with bilateral proximal radio-ulnar joint synostosis. Right forearm fused in neutral and left fixed in slight pronation. (*Courtesy of Shriners Hospital for Children, Philadelphia, PA; with permission.*)

Mild degrees of fixed pronation or supination are well tolerated and require no treatment.[2] Extremes of position create functional difficulties and may require rotational osteotomy through the fusion mass to a more functional position (**Fig. 9**).[6–8] Treatment strategies aimed at restoration of motion are universally unsuccessful and are not recommended. Caution must be used with severe rotational deformities to prevent a neurovascular complication.

Preoperative evaluation The optimal rotational position of the forearm is controversial, because the best position varies with the task. A preoperative evaluation by an occupational therapist helps determine the individual child's functional deficits and optimal forearm position. Bilateral recommendations are to place the dominant forearm in 10° to 20° of pronation and the nondominant forearm in neutral rotation.[8]

Unilateral recommendations are to position the forearm in slight pronation, as 30° of pronation provides the best function for writing and working with small objects.

Surgical technique: osteotomy The child is positioned supine and the arm is placed on a table. A pediatric tourniquet is placed high on the arm to position the epicondylar axis within the surgical field for accurate measurement of forearm rotation. A longitudinal dorsal incision is made over the synostosis along the subcutaneous border of the ulna between the extensor carpi ulnaris and the flexor carpi ulnaris (**Fig. 10**). Sharp dissection is performed directly on the synostosis. Avoid proximal exposure that will enter the elbow joint and avoid too distal an exposure that will miss the synostosis. Reverse or bent malleable retractors are placed around the synostosis. Avoid excessive traction on the retractors, which can injure the posterior interosseous and ulnar nerves.

A wire driver is used to place a smooth Steinman pin .062 in from a percutaneous position through the olecranon epiphysis into the intramedullary canal of the ulna (**Fig. 11**). The pin is positioned just proximal to the planned osteotomy site. Mini-fluoroscopy is helpful to ensure correct placement. The longitudinal alignment of the forearm is marked before osteotomy to assess the degree of rotation after osteotomy. A transverse osteotomy is performed through the fusion mass with an oscillating saw under direct vision and irrigation (**Fig. 12**). The osteotomy must be complete because incomplete osteotomy can leave a bony spike that prohibits rotation and bony alignment.

The forearm is rotated into the desired position. The longitudinal wire is advanced across the osteotomy site. An additional percutaneous oblique Kirschner wire is placed across the osteotomy for rotational control (**Fig. 13**). The pins are left in

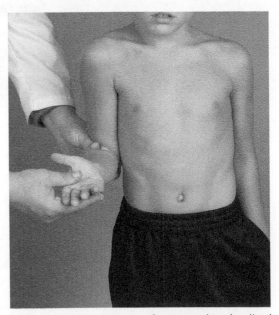

Fig. 5. Forearm motion must be assessed at the distal radioulnar joint to avoid false interpretation of forearm movement. (*Courtesy of Shriners Hospital for Children, Philadelphia, PA; with permission.*)

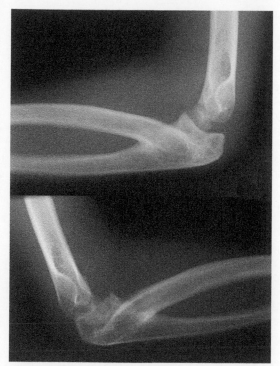

Fig. 6. Radiographs confirm bilateral proximal radioulnar joint synostosis. (*Courtesy of* Shriners Hospital for Children, Philadelphia, PA; with permission.)

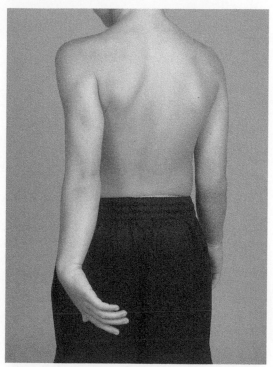

Fig. 8. Lack of supination creates difficulty with toileting. (*Courtesy of* Shriners Hospital for Children, Philadelphia, PA; with permission.)

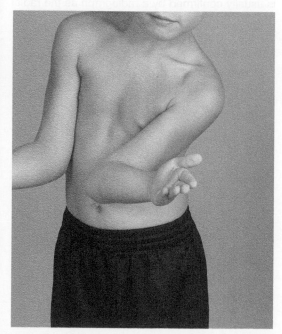

Fig. 7. Shoulder adduction compensates for deficient supination. (*Courtesy of* Shriners Hospital for Children, Philadelphia, PA; with permission.)

a percutaneous position. The subcutaneous tissue and skin are closed with an absorbable suture. Avoid closing the fascia, as this may increase the possibility of a compartment syndrome. The arm is placed in a long arm cast with the elbow flexed to 90°. The child is admitted to the hospital overnight for strict elevation and neurovascular monitoring.

The cast and pins are removed in the office after bony union, usually 6 weeks after surgery (**Fig. 14**). Early active motion is encouraged. Children usually regain elbow and wrist motion without therapy.

Radial head dislocation

Radial head dislocation can occur in isolation or is associated with proximal radioulnar synostosis (**Fig. 15**). Radial head dislocation is associated with numerous other syndromes, such as Klinefelter, trisomy 13, Cornelia de Lange, Ehlers-Danlos, and nail-patella syndrome.[1] The direction of dislocation is usually posterior or posterolateral in approximately two thirds of the cases. Anterior dislocation occurs in approximately one third of the cases.[9–11] Congenital radial head dislocation often presents after a perceived elbow injury and may be erroneously attributed to that injury. A unilateral, congenital radial head dislocation may be difficult to distinguish from chronic traumatic

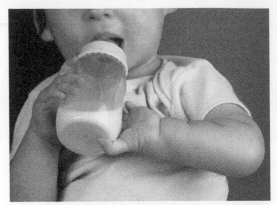

Fig. 9. A 1-year-old child with left proximal radioulnar joint synostosis and extreme pronation that prohibits bringing left hand to mouth. (*Courtesy of* Shriners Hospital for Children, Philadelphia, PA; with permission.)

dislocation. Radiographic criteria that support a congenital dislocation include a short radius (relative to the ulna), hypoplastic capitellum with a deficient trochlea, and a dome-shaped radial head (**Fig. 16**).[10,11] However these findings can also develop as a result of a traumatic dislocation at an early age. Family history and bilateral involvement also infer a congenital cause.

The presenting complaint in a posterior or posterolateral dislocation is usually a prominent posterolateral bone (ie, the radial head), restricted

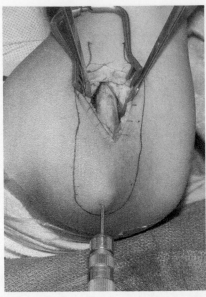

Fig. 11. Steinman pin inserted through the olecranon apophysis and into the intramedullary canal of the ulna. (*Courtesy of* Shriners Hospital for Children, Philadelphia, PA; with permission.)

elbow extension (usually terminal 30°), and decreased forearm rotation (about one-half normal) (**Fig. 17**). An anterior dislocated radial head presents with a prominence in the antecubital fossa, deficient terminal elbow flexion, and mildly decreased forearm rotation. The diagnosis is usually confirmed by a radiograph as the radial

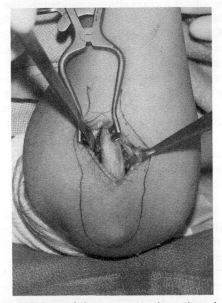

Fig. 10. Exposure of the synostosis along the subcutaneous border of the ulna between extensor carpi ulnaris and the flexor carpi ulnaris. (*Courtesy of* Shriners Hospital for Children, Philadelphia, PA; with permission.)

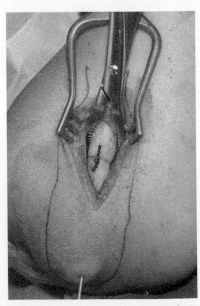

Fig. 12. Transverse osteotomy through the fusion mass. (*Courtesy of* Shriners Hospital for Children, Philadelphia, PA; with permission.)

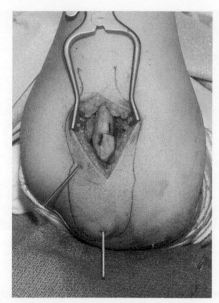

Fig. 13. The forearm is rotated and the longitudinal wire is advanced across the osteotomy site. An additional percutaneous oblique Kirschner wire is placed across the osteotomy for rotational control. (*Courtesy of* Shriners Hospital for Children, Philadelphia, PA; with permission.)

head fails to align with the capitellum. Additional radiograph findings include dysplasia of the capitellum with loss of the anterior humeral line, abnormal shape of the radial head, and ulnar positive variance.[10,11] In the infant, the unossified dislocated radial head may be visualized with advanced imaging studies, such as magnetic resonance imaging or diagnostic ultrasound.[12]

Treatment is seldom necessary in childhood. Most children are asymptomatic and have minimal functional limitations. Open reduction with annular ligament reconstruction has not been consistently successful.[1,13,14] In adolescence or adulthood, a dislocated radial head may become painful because of degenerative changes at the contact point between the radial head and the capitellum.

Excision of the radial head will alleviate symptoms.[10]

Surgical technique: radial head resection The adolescent is positioned supine and the arm is placed across the chest or on a table. A tourniquet is placed high on the arm. Previously, we used a Kocher approach between the extensor carpi ulnaris and the anconeus for radial head exposure. This approach, however, jeopardizes the lateral collateral ligament of the elbow and can result in posterolateral instability. The current approach is straight lateral just anterior to the lateral epicondyle and extending over the radial head (**Fig. 18**). The forearm fascia is incised and the extensor digitorum muscle fibers are split. A longitudinal arthrotomy is performed to expose the radial head and neck.

In children with an anteriorly dislocated radial head, the surgical exposure is more difficult and the posterior interosseous nerve is in more jeopardy. If in doubt about the location of the posterior interosseous nerve, I use an anterior approach to locate and protect the nerve before radial head excision.

Once the posteriorly dislocated radial head is isolated, the forearm is pronated to protect the posterior interosseous nerve. Reverse retractors

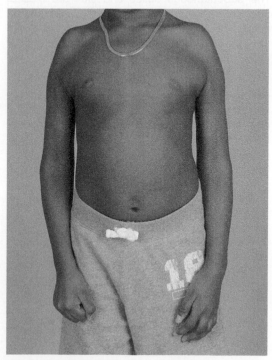

Fig. 15. A 7-year-old child with bilateral posterolateral radial head dislocations. (*Courtesy of* Shriners Hospital for Children, Philadelphia, PA; with permission.)

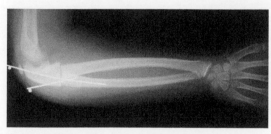

Fig. 14. Radiographs after rotational osteotomy with good fixation. (*Courtesy of* Shriners Hospital for Children, Philadelphia, PA; with permission.)

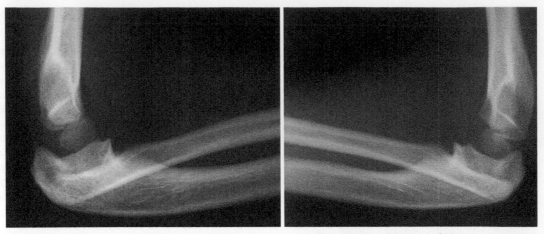

Fig. 16. Radiographs reveal bilateral posterolateral radial head dislocations. (*Courtesy of* Shriners Hospital for Children, Philadelphia, PA; with permission.)

are placed around the radial neck. The radial head is excised with a saw perpendicular to the radial neck (**Fig. 19**). The radial head is removed (**Fig. 20**). The elbow is moved through a full range of motion to make sure that the proximal radius does not contact the distal humerus. Additional impingement requires further resection. Bone wax is applied to the radial neck. The capsule is closed with a nonabsorbable suture (**Fig. 21**). The subcutaneous tissue and skin are closed. Local anesthesia is used for postoperative analgesia. The arm is placed in a long arm splint with the elbow at 90° for 7 to 10 days, followed by active motion. Formal therapy is usually not necessary.

Outcome and complications Radial head excision reliably relieves pain, improves appearance, and may improve range of motion.[10,15,16] Complications include regrowth of the proximal radius, posterior interosseous nerve injury, and cubitus valgus deformity.[15,16] In 25 children who

underwent radial head resection for a variety of reasons, however, cubitus valgus was not found during follow-up at an average age of 14 years (range 5 to 18 years).[16]

Arthrogryposis

Arthrogryposis or congenital multiple arthrogryposis is a syndrome of joint contractures that are present at birth and nonprogressive.[17] There are multiple forms of arthrogryposis that vary in presentation, severity, and number of involved joints. In addition, there are a multitude of syndromes and genetic conditions that have features of arthrogryposis. A classic example is Freeman-Sheldon syndrome (also known as whistling face syndrome), an autosomal dominant condition affecting the hands and feet with a characteristic facial appearance.[18] Another example is Beals syndrome, an inheritable condition with contractural arachnodactyly, proximal interphalangeal joint flexion contractures, and a characteristic

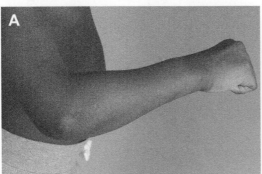
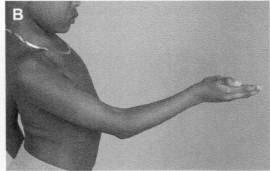

Fig. 17. Presenting signs of posterolateral radial head dislocation. (*A*) Prominent radial head. (*B*) Lack of full elbow extension and restricted forearm supination. (*Courtesy of* Shriners Hospital for Children, Philadelphia, PA; with permission.)

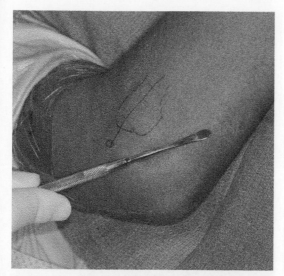

Fig. 18. Lateral incision just anterior to the lateral epicondyle and extending in a distal direction over the radial head. Freer elevator indicates Kocher interval between the extensor carpi ulnaris and the anconeus straight. (*Courtesy of* Shriners Hospital for Children, Philadelphia, PA; with permission.)

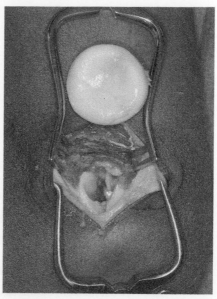

Fig. 20. Radial head removed after osteotomy of radial neck. (*Courtesy of* Shriners Hospital for Children, Philadelphia, PA; with permission.)

"crumpled" ear.[19] The windblown hand (also known as congenital ulnar drift) is also a variation of arthrogryposis and is usually inherited as an autosomal dominant trait.[20]

The elbow is frequently the most problematic joint in children with arthrogryposis.[21–23] The elbow is usually contracted in full extension. Lack of flexion prohibits hand-to-mouth function and many daily tasks. The first goal is restoration of passive motion. Adequate passive flexion allows the hand to be placed near the face using a tabletop or adaptive equipment (**Fig. 22**). Early efforts to restore passive elbow flexion are critical and are emphasized in therapy. Recalcitrant elbow extension requires consideration for surgical

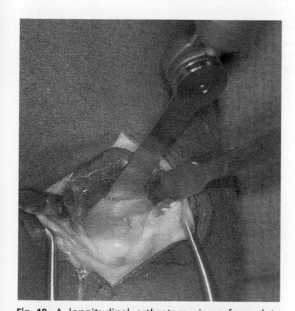

Fig. 19. A longitudinal arthrotomy is performed to expose the radial head and neck. The radial head is excised with a saw perpendicular to the radial neck straight. (*Courtesy of* Shriners Hospital for Children, Philadelphia, PA; with permission.)

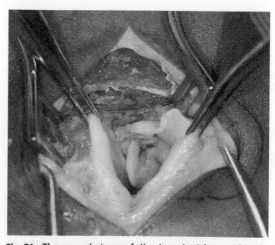

Fig. 21. The capsule is carefully closed with nonabsorbable suture. (*Courtesy of* Shriners Hospital for Children, Philadelphia, PA; with permission.)

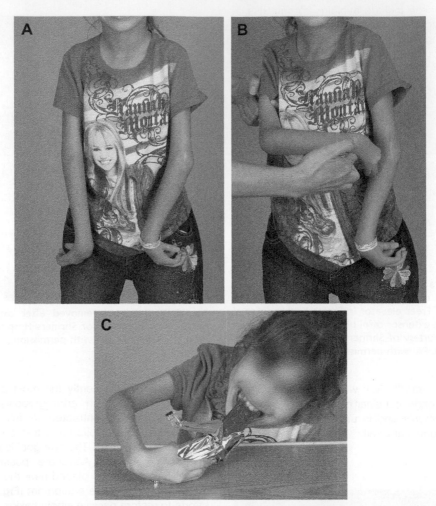

Fig. 22. A 7-year-old child with arthrogryposis and passive right elbow flexion, but no active elbow flexion. (*A*) Upright posture with elbows extended. (*B*) Passive right elbow flexion. (*C*) Passive elbow flexion via table top and wrist flexion for eating. (*Courtesy of* Shriners Hospital for Children, Philadelphia, PA; with permission.)

release by lengthening of the triceps and posterior capsular release.[22]

A secondary goal is restoration of active elbow flexion.[23] Passive flexion is a prerequisite to active motion. Potential donor muscles for elbow flexor-plasty include the pectoralis major, latissimus dorsi, triceps, and flexor-pronator mass.[23,24] The available donor muscle must be expendable and possess adequate strength and excursion. The selection of donor muscle is more difficult in children with arthrogryposis. Adequate evaluation of muscle strength is difficult in children and excursion is often lacking. Furthermore, potential donor muscles may be contraindicated. For example, triceps transfer is contraindicated in children who use upper extremity devices (eg, crutches) to ambulate. Unfortunately, the results after elbow flexion transfers for arthrogryposis are not as

predictable compared with other causes.[23] This inconsistent outcome reflects the lack of passive joint motion, the paucity of donor muscles, and the inadequate quality of the donor muscle.

Surgical technique: posterior release
A posterior surgical approach is used by way of a curvilinear incision that extends over the medial aspect of the elbow. The ulnar nerve is transposed from the cubital tunnel into a subcutaneous position. The triceps is lengthened as long as possible using a V-to-Y technique. The triceps is reflected to reveal the posterior capsule, which is divided form medial to lateral. The elbow is flexed with an ultimate goal of greater than 90° of flexion. Forceful flexion is not applied to avoid damaging the distal humerus growth plate. The triceps is approximated in a V-to-Y method. The wound is closed and the

arm splinted in full flexion for 3 weeks. A splint is fabricated at 90° of flexion and passive elbow flexion initiated. Activities that require elbow flexion are encouraged. Some elbow extension strength will return depending upon the integrity of the triceps muscle and tendon.

Pterygium

A pterygium or web across the antecubital fossa can occur in isolation or as part of a syndrome (**Fig. 23**). Associated syndromes include multiple pterygium syndrome, thrombocytopenia absent radius, and multiple synostosis syndrome. The pterygium is a harbinger of underlying abnormalities that occurred in utero and all of those abnormalities prohibit elbow extension. Simple release, lengthening, or replacement of the pterygium will have negligible effect on improving elbow extension. Extensive elbow release and application of distraction devices have also been disappointing. Currently, nonoperative management is the main treatment by prescribing occupational therapy and adaptive equipment to facilitate self-care and activities of daily living.

CONGENITAL DIFFERENCES THAT AFFECT ELBOW MOTION AND STABILITY OVER TIME

The forearm joint is a paired bone structure that provides pronation and supination. The radius and ulna are held together by the proximal radioulnar joint, interosseous membrane, and the distal radioulnar joint. The forearm joint also functions in force transmission from the wrist to the elbow. Although there is some debate as to exact amount, the radius carries the majority of the load at the wrist (radiocarpal joint) and the ulna supports the preponderance of the load at the elbow (ulnohumeral joint).[25–27] The load is transferred from the radius to the ulna by way of the interosseous membrane. This transfer requires an intact interosseous membrane and similar lengths of the radius and ulna. Any condition that affects the length of the radius or ulna will disrupt this load transmission across the forearm. There are many traumatic, acquired, or congenital conditions that directly impair the growth of the radius and ulna. Physeal injuries, infections, compartment syndromes, and tumors are examples of traumatic and acquired causes. Multiple hereditary exostosis, multiple enchondromas (Ollier disease), skeletal dysplasia, and osteogenesis imperfecta are examples of congenital causes that commonly disturb forearm integrity.

Multiple Hereditary Exostosis

Multiple hereditary exostosis (MHE) tends to affect the distal ulna more than the radius, which leads to ulnar shortening. This length inequality changes the normal load propagation across the forearm. The radius bears all load at the wrist and a greater load through the forearm, as the force transfer across the interosseous membrane lessens. The growing radius adapts to the intensive load by

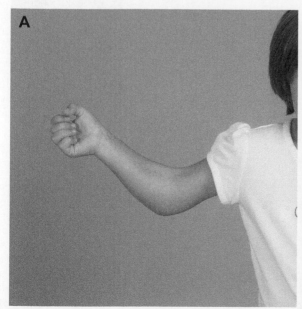
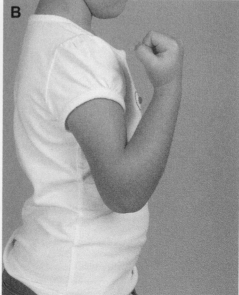

Fig. 23. A 7-year-old child with isolated right elbow pterygium. (*A*) Deficient elbow extension. (*B*) Good elbow flexion. (*Courtesy of* Shriners Hospital for Children, Philadelphia, PA; with permission.)

tilting of the articular surface, hypertrophy, and bowing. However, the radiocapitellar joint is poorly designed for this type of load bearing. In some cases, the radius bows to a point and the radiocapitellar joint remains located (**Fig. 24**). In other cases, the radial head subluxates or dislocates depending upon the magnitude of the load and restraining properties of the proximal radioulnar joint. The ideal treatment would restore forearm anatomy and load transmission.

The decision to intervene in MHE is difficult and controversial. Early osteochondroma removal to prevent or retard progressive growth disturbances is debatable.[28] In addition, two studies reveal that adults with untreated forearm deformities due to MHE maintained their function and were comfortable with their appearance.[29,30] These studies question the role of surgical treatment to maintain or improve function. However, MHE has an extremely variable phenotype and children with severe cases have countless number of exostosis and substantial deformity.

Decisive treatment factors include forearm motion, interval change, degree of ulnar shortening, status of the radiocapitellar joint, preference of the family, and the surgeon's philosophy. My operative indications include progressive motion loss, radial head subluxation, and ongoing ulnar shortening. Contraindications include a mild

deformity with good motion and a stable forearm in a skeletally mature individual. In children with progressive ulnar shortening and radial head subluxation, ulnar lengthening is performed to restore the normal forearm framework. Ulnar lengthening can be done by way of a single stage Z-lengthening or by using distraction osteogenesis and an external fixator. I prefer distraction osteogenesis using a uniplane lengthening device. If a concomitant angular deformity is present, an acute angular correction can be performed at the time of external fixator application or a multiplanar external fixator can be applied and the angulation slowly corrected. The goal is to slightly overlengthen the ulna and restore forearm anatomy. Restoration of normal forearm anatomy will prevent radial head subluxation and can result in spontaneous radial head reduction.

In children with severe radial inclination, correction can be obtained by radial osteotomy or hemi-epiphyseal stapling of the radial side of the distal radius in the young child. This retards radial growth and allows correction of the radial articular angle with growth.[31] Osteotomy or stapling can be performed in conjunction with ulnar lengthening.

Surgical technique: uniplanar external fixation
The ulna is exposed over its subcutaneous border between the flexor carpi ulnaris and the extensor

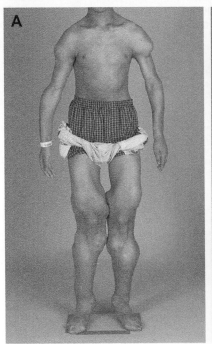
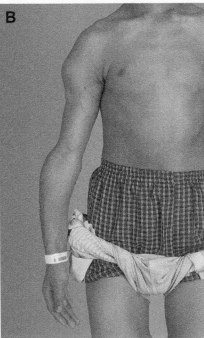
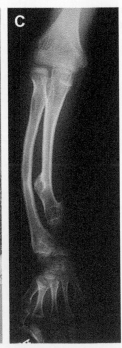

Fig. 24. A 16-year-old male with severe MHE. (*A*) Upper and lower extremities are severely involved. (*B*) Bowing of right forearm. (*C*) Radiographs show ulnar shortening and radial bowing. Radiocapitellar joint is located. (*Courtesy of* Shriners Hospital for Children, Philadelphia, PA; with permission.)

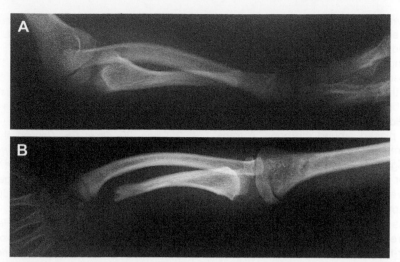

Fig. 25. An 8-year-old child with shortened left forearm after infection (*A*) Anteroposterior radiograph shows loss of distal ulna, growth plate arrest, and radial bowing. (*B*) Lateral radiographs reveal radial head dislocation. (*Courtesy of* Shriners Hospital for Children, Philadelphia, PA; with permission.)

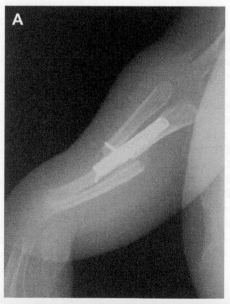

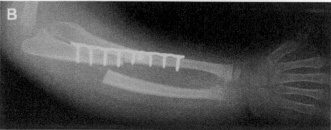

Fig. 26. One-bone forearm after transposition of distal radius onto proximal ulna along with radial head resection. (*A*) Anteroposterior radiograph shows stable forearm after rigid fixation with remaining radius used as on-lay graft. (*B*) Lateral radiograph confirms adequate radial head resection and acceptable forearm alignment. (*Courtesy of* Shriners Hospital for Children, Philadelphia, PA; with permission.)

carpi ulnaris leaving the periosteum intact. The appropriately sized uniplanar external fixator is selected based on the size of the ulna and the anticipated lengthening necessary. The external fixator is applied using a standard technique with two bicortical threaded pins placed proximal and distal to the proposed osteotomy site. The periosteum is elevated at the osteotomy site and reverse retractors are placed around the bone. A transverse osteotomy is performed using a saw and continuous irrigation to limit bone necrosis. The external fixator is distracted until the bone separates to ensure complete osteotomy. The bony ends are reapproximated and the skin is closed. Lengthening is started 7 to 10 days later, at 1 mm/d, and requires careful follow-up. The ulna is slightly over-lengthened. The external fixator is removed after adequate bony consolidation shown by radiograph.

If a concomitant angular deformity is present, an acute angular correction is performed before external fixator application. This osteotomy prevents provisional fixator application and requires careful planning.

The Unsalvageable Forearm

Formation of a one-bone forearm may be used to salvage a severely disorganized forearm secondary to MHE, Ollier disease, or bone loss (**Fig. 25**).[32] This procedure provides immediate stability to the forearm. A dislocated radial head can be removed at the same time. The incisions must be carefully planned and the neurovascular structures vigilantly protected. I prefer to transpose the distal radius onto the proximal ulna and to obtain rigid fixation (**Fig. 26**). This technique preserves the distal radius and proximal ulna growth plates. In addition, the radius cut is performed distal to the ulnar cut. After transposition, the remaining proximal radius is used as an onlay graft to promote union.

SUMMARY

The elbow is frequently affected by congenital differences that limit flexion–extension and supination–pronation. The limitation can occur in utero or develop over time. Delayed causes usually gradually disrupt the anatomy and function of the paired bone forearm. Accurate diagnosis is based on a careful examination and perusal of radiographs. Certain diagnoses can be helped by surgery and will result in improved limb usage and function. In contrast, other diagnoses are recalcitrant to modern operative techniques, but will benefit from occupational therapy and adaptive equipment to enhance independence and activities essential to daily life.

REFERENCES

1. Kozin SH. Upper-extremity congenital anomalies. Current concepts review. J Bone Joint Surg Am 2003;85:1564–75.
2. Cleary JE, Omer GE. Congenital proximal radioulnar synostosis: natural history and functional assessment. J Bone Joint Surg Am 1985;67:539–45.
3. Hansen OH, Andersen NO. Congenital radio-ulnar synostosis. Report of 37 cases. Acta Orthop Scand 1970;41:225–30.
4. Edwards MJ, Rowe L, Petroff V. Herrmann multiple synostosis syndrome with neurological complications caused by spinal canal stenosis. Am J Med Genet 2000;95:118–22.
5. Ogino T, Hikino K. Congenital radio-ulnar synostosis: compensatory rotation around the wrist and rotation osteotomy. J Hand Surg [Br] 1987;12:173–8.
6. Simmons BP, Southmayd WW, Riseborough EJ. Congenital radioulnar synostosis. J Hand Surg [Am] 1983;8:829–38.
7. Bolano LE. Congenital proximal radioulnar synostosis: treatment with the Ilizarov method. J Hand Surg [Am] 1994;19:977–8.
8. Green WT, Mital MA. Congenital radio-ulnar synostosis: surgical treatment. J Bone Joint Surg Am 1979;61:738–43.
9. Mardam-Bey TE, Ger E. Congenital radial head dislocation. J Hand Surg 1979;4:316–20.
10. Kelly DW. Congenital dislocation of the radial head: spectrum and natural history. J Pediatr Orthop 1981; 1:295–8.
11. Agnew DK, Davis RJ. Congenital unilateral dislocation of the radial head. J Pediatr Orthop 1993;13: 526–8.
12. Bar-On EC, Howard B, Porat S. The use of ultrasound in the diagnosis of atypical pathology in the unossified skeleton. J Pediatr Orthop 1995;15:817–20.
13. Miura T. Congenital dislocation of the radial head. J Hand Surg [Br] 1990;15:477–81.
14. Sachar K, Mih AD. Congenital radial head dislocations. Hand Clin 1998;14:39–47.
15. Campbell CC, Waters PM, Emans JB. Excision of the radial head for congenital dislocation. J Bone Joint Surg Am 1992;74:726–33.
16. Hresko MT, Rosenberg BN, Pappas AM. Excision of the radial head in patients younger than 18 years. J Pediatr Orthop 1999;19:106–13.
17. Hall JG, Reed SD, Driscoll EP. Part I. Amyoplasia: a common, sporadic condition with congenital contractures. Am J Med Genet 1983;15:571–90.
18. Krakowiak PA, Bohnsack JF, Carey JC, et al. Clinical analysis of a variant of Freeman-Sheldon syndrome (DA2B). Am J Med Genet 1998;76:93–8.

19. Beals RK, Hecht F. Congenital contractural arachnodactyly. A heritable disorder of connective tissue. J Bone Joint Surg Am 1971;53:987–93.

20. Bamshad M, Bohnsack JF, Jorde LB, et al. Distal arthrogryposis type 1: clinical analysis of a large kindred. Am J Med Genet 1996;65:282–5.

21. Bennett JB, Hansen PE, Granberry WM, et al. Surgical management of arthrogryposis of the upper extremity. J Pediatr Orthop 1985;5:281–6.

22. Ezaki M. Treatment of the upper limb in the child with arthrogryposis. Hand Clin 2000;16:703–11.

23. Van Heest A, Waters PM, Simmons BP. Surgical treatment of arthrogryposis of the elbow. J Hand Surg [Am] 1998;23:1063–70.

24. Kozin SH. Injuries of the brachial plexus. In: Iannotti JP, Williams GR, editors. Disorders of the shoulder: diagnosis and management. Philadelphia: Lippincott Williams & Wilkins; 1999. p. 847–80.

25. Birbeck DP, Failla JM, Hoshaw SJ, et al. The interosseous membrane affects load distribution in the forearm. J Hand Surg [Am] 1997;22:975–80.

26. McGinley JC, Heller JE, Fertala A, et al. Biomechanical composition and histologic structure of the forearm interosseous membrane. J Hand Surg [Am] 2003;28:503–10.

27. Hotchkiss RN, An KN, Sowa DT, et al. An anatomic and mechanical study of the interosseous membrane of the forearm: pathomechanics of proximal migration of the radius. J Hand Surg [Am] 1989;14A: 256–61.

28. Masada K, Tsuyuguchi Y, Kawai H, et al. Operations for forearm deformity caused by multiple osteochondromas. J Bone Joint Surg Br 1989;71:24–9.

29. Stanton RP, Hansen MO. Function of the upper extremities in hereditary multiple exostoses. J Bone Joint Surg Am 1996;78:568–73.

30. Arms DM, Strecker WB, Manske PR, et al. Management of forearm deformity in multiple hereditary osteochondromatosis. J Pediatr Orthop 1997;17:450–4.

31. Wood VE, Sauser D, Mudge D. The treatment of hereditary multiple exostosis of the upper extremity. J Hand Surg [Am] 1985;10:505–13.

32. Rodgers WB, Hall JE. One-bone forearm as a salvage procedure for recalcitrant forearm deformity in hereditary multiple exostoses. J Pediatr Orthop 1993;13:587–91.

Congenital Hand Surgery: What's New and What's Coming

Charles A. Goldfarb, MD

KEYWORDS

- Longitudinal deficiency • Syndactyly • Polydactyly
- Apert's syndrome • Toe transfer • Callotasis

Progress in our understanding of congenital hand anomalies has been steady over the last decade with retrospective reports on diagnosis, classification, and treatment strategies found in multiple journals. The platform of any discussion of future advancements in hand surgery is a review of the current state, specifically including recent advancements in the field. To assess the current state of congenital hand surgery, the author has reviewed the content of the last 12 years from seven journals including: *The Journal of Pediatric Orthopedics*, *The Journal of Hand Surgery* (American and British), *The Journal of Bone and Joint Surgery* (American and British), *Plastic and Reconstructive Surgery*, and *Hand Surgery*. These journals are multispecialty, represent the worldwide hand surgery community, and all publish articles pertinent to the topic of congenital hand surgery. There were fewer than 110 articles on congenital hand surgery identified in the initial search and, after eliminating case reports, technique articles, review articles, and some smaller scientific articles, 70 articles were reviewed in more depth. A smaller number still was chosen to represent the progress made in congenital hand surgery over these years. This review is strictly limited to congenital hand surgery and, therefore, the tangentially related topics of cerebral palsy, arthrogryposis, birth brachial plexus palsy, multiple hereditary exostosis, and Madelung's deformity are excluded.

The number of pertinent articles identified (approximately six per year total) is surprisingly low for a survey of these seven journals. Most of the articles are retrospective assessments of a particular congenital hand abnormality. Although these reports are helpful, the study type and the typically small numbers of patients included provide for only incremental progress in our understanding of these conditions. Prospective trials have been limited due to the rarity of the diagnoses and the difficulty of conducting multicenter trials. However, the future of congenital hand surgery is exciting, primarily because of the hope of greater understanding through molecular genetics and translational research. Our improved understanding of the genetics and pathways of normal, and therefore abnormal, development should allow improved classification schemes and, eventually, intervention to prevent, modify, or remedy these birth abnormalities.

BENCHTOP RESEARCH

The article of Isogai and colleagues[1] stands out in its reporting of the formation of phalanges and joints from tissue engineering techniques with the use of periosteum, chondrocytes, and tenocytes in a biodegradable synthetic polymer scaffold. The concept of using tissue engineering to create bones and joints has been discussed for years; this investigation provides evidence that the technique is possible, albeit still in the future for routine clinical use.

Naruse and colleagues[2] reported on the administration of bulsulfan in rats in an effort to understand the relationship between central deficiency, polydactyly, and syndactyly. The authors evaluated the embryos at days 12 to 21 and found

Department of Orthopaedic Surgery, Washington University School of Medicine at Barnes Jewish Hospital, 660 South Euclid Avenue, Campus Box 8233, St Louis, MO 63110, USA
E-mail address: goldfarbc@wudosis.wustl.edu

Hand Clin 25 (2009) 293–299
doi:10.1016/j.hcl.2008.10.006
0749-0712/08/$ – see front matter © 2009 Elsevier Inc. All rights reserved.

that similar abnormal clefts in the embryos accounted for the development of all three abnormalities. The authors concluded that these abnormalities should be classified as a single category- abnormal induction of digital rays.

There have been numerous advances in our understanding of molecular biology and molecular genetics; the progress of the Human Genome Project sets the stage for the rapid progress of our understanding of normal and abnormal development. The extent of our improved understanding is made clear through the *Online Mendelian Inheritance in Man* Web site (part of the US National Library of Medicine and National Institutes of Health), which cites the single gene mutations responsible for numerous congenital abnormalities. These reports are too numerous to mention, but each is important in our march toward understanding development. The progress toward identification of the single gene mutations responsible for these disorders is exciting and will continue at an even more rapid rate in the near future. The future is also promising for gene therapy as a tool to correct single gene disorders and to assist in the management of other health abnormalities.[3]

CLASSIFICATION

In the current state, our classification algorithms remain rooted in a descriptive and treatment-based hierarchy and notable contributions have been made to clarify the classification system over the last decade. James and colleagues[4] demonstrated that radial longitudinal deficiency (RLD) represents a spectrum of abnormalities from thumb hypoplasia alone to the complete absence of the radius. A modification of the Bayne and Klug classification system was suggested to incorporate isolated thumb hypoplasia and a deficiency of the radial carpus to RLD classification.[5]

A re-examination of the concept of phocomelia suggested that, in most cases, it is not truly an intercalary defect.[6] In a review of 44 extremities diagnosed with phocomelia, 33 were considered not to be an intercalary deficiency after additional review. Another article concluded that most patients with a diagnosis of phocomelia instead have a longitudinal deficiency that represents a severe manifestation of either RLD or ulnar longitudinal deficiency (ULD).[7] Those patients with a severe RLD may have an absent proximal humerus whereas those with a severe ULD typically present with a single long bone for the upper extremity that may bifurcate distally.

As our understanding of the human genome progresses, we are beginning to identify the genetic abnormalities that are responsible for some of the common upper extremity congenital anomalies. It is inevitable that our classification system will be altered to incorporate the genetic etiology of these disorders. It is interesting to ponder, as hand surgeons, this concept of a genetically-based classification. We are taught that classification systems should help us to better understand a problem and provide guidance for the treatment of the problem. When we truly understand the genetics of upper extremity abnormalities, a new classification system will emerge that will explain the etiology of the abnormality (genetic locus of abnormality, timing of insult, and so forth) and, eventually, allow treatment through gene therapy or other intervention. This shift in classification and treatment is closer than ever but certainly is still many years away.

RADIAL LONGITUDINAL DEFICIENCY

Four recent articles provide the long-term outcome of RLD treated with a centralization procedure.[8–11] While surgical technique and outcome assessment differed among the articles, the key message from all four was that the deformity will recur after centralization. All reported that the degree of the initial deformity is the most important factor in recurrence, whereas the specifics of the surgical technique (ie, whether to notch the distal ulna) contribute less to the risk of recurrence. Hand function remained decreased after centralization. However, upper extremity function, as assessed by the disabilities of the arm, shoulder, and hand outcome questionnaire, was only mildly affected; perhaps due to the ability of the affected to accommodate to their given limb. One benefit of the centralization procedure is that it places the hand on the end of the ulna; this improves the aesthetic appearance of the extremity by the additional length and decreased deformity. However, the centralization procedure may affect ulnar growth, especially if the ulna is aggressively notched or if there is a high degree of tension needed to place the hand on the end of the ulna. A recent investigation examined ulnar growth patterns and found that the ulna achieved 64% of expected length in nonoperated patients, 58% of normal length in patients centralized without notching, and 48% of normal length in patients with a notched distal ulna at centralization.[12] So, while centralization can place the hand on the end of the ulna to provide additional length to the extremity, ulna growth-plate injury should be avoided by less forceful reduction of the carpus.

Two recently described techniques address the shortcomings of centralization. First, Vilkki[13] reported the 6-year follow-up on patients with RLD treated with microvascular transfer of the second metatarsophalangeal joint to the radial side of the wrist joint after soft-tissue distraction. This innovative technique provides a mobile joint to support the radial wrist but it is technically challenging. Three articles reported results of ring fixator distraction of the soft tissues before centralization.[14–16] The technique of gradual soft tissue distraction makes the centralization procedure much easier (and safer) technically and allows a more balanced reconstruction. Long-term results on recurrence are needed to evaluate the hypothesis that the more balanced initial reconstruction will lead to a decreased risk of recurrence.

Lengthening of the forearm has been used in two ways in RLD. First, in patients with type II or III RLD, the radius may be lengthened to help balance the wrist. This technique may require soft-tissue releases and multiple lengthening procedures as the child grows, with hopes to maintain wrist motion and alignment.[17] If the radius and ulna lengths are equal (type 0 RLD) or equalized after lengthening of the radius, the patient may be treated effectively with dorsal tendon balancing surgery with a good expected outcome.[18]

The second use of callotasis is for lengthening of the ulna that may allow a more normal appearance and function of the extremity.[19,20] Complete consolidation after Ilizarov lengthening may take longer than expected, but up to a 50% increase in length may be accomplished. Complications including infection are also common. Horii and colleagues[21] reported on a mixed group of patients treated with forearm distraction lengthening; there was a higher incidence of complications in congenital cases but a satisfactory 35% length increase was accomplished.

Finally, multiple comorbidities may affect patients with RLD. Cardiac abnormalities, spinal abnormalities, and lower-extremity musculoskeletal abnormalities are all common. Thrombocytopenia-Absent Radius Syndrome and vertebral, anal, cardiac, tracheoesophageal, renal, and limb abnormality association were the most common syndromic associations. In the initial evaluation of a patient with RLD, a thorough history and physical examination should be performed and additional testing, including cardiac and renal ultrasound, spinal radiographs, and blood work (complete blood count and genetic testing for Fanconi's anemia) has been suggested.[22]

HYPOPLASTIC THUMB

One article reviewed 15 pollicization procedures with greater than 20-year follow-up. Ten of the pollicized digits were used as normal thumbs. The authors concluded that satisfactory long-term functional and aesthetic results can be expected.[23] Another investigation reported on a comprehensive treatment approach for the Blauth type IIIA, pollux abductus thumb.[24] The authors recommended an extensile exposure of the thumb to the forearm to identify and treat tendinous and muscular interconnections between the flexor and extensor tendons. Opposition transfer was performed in eight of the thumbs, and treatment of the thumb-index web space and the metacarpophalangeal joint stability were performed as needed. This more comprehensive approach to the pollux abductus was felt to offer the best chance at improved function.

Another investigation compared four patients with Blauth type IIIB thumbs reconstructed using vascularized metatarsophalangeal joint with other patients treated with pollicization.[25] While the pollicized digits were more normal appearing, function (as assessed by strength and dexterity) was better in the reconstructed group. The authors concluded that reconstruction is a viable alternative to pollicization. Finally, the objective features of pollicized digits in a large number of patients were assessed subjectively and objectively compared against age-matched normals.[26] Decreased girth, excess length, and angulation were the most notable abnormalities.

ULNAR LONGITUDINAL DEFICIENCY

Three articles offer advances in our understanding of ULD through a more comprehensive classification of these abnormalities. The first describes a classification based on the degree of deficiency of the thumb and first web space.[27] This classification of the radial hand is helpful from a practical perspective because most surgery in ULD is targeted to the hand abnormalities, not the abnormalities of the forearm. The second article presents 13 extremities with ULD isolated to the hand (normal ulna length); abnormalities in these cases include ulnar-sided ectrodactyly and metacarpal synostosis with a normal forearm.[28] This suggests that, as in RLD, there may be ULD confined to the hand. The final article describes the clinical findings in type IV ULD.[29] Findings among the patients were highly variable and surgical intervention was not always required; when performed, surgery was often on the hand.

CONGENITAL BELOW-ELBOW AMPUTATION

The results of a multicenter outcomes study on unilateral congenital below-elbow amputation

(BEA) are beginning to be published. In one report it was concluded that, based on an assessment of 489 children (prosthesis wearers or nonwearers), prostheses do not help to improve function or quality of life.[30] This is an important finding because it calls into question the common practice of early prosthesis fitting. Other findings from this study are pending. Another investigation from a single institution found that fitting a prosthesis at less than 3 years old, the provision of intensive training in prosthetic wear, and the availability of different prosthetic designs with growth all significantly helped support the success of early fitting.[31] While the messages from these important investigation seems mixed, the importance of a comprehensive assessment, a thorough education of the family, and, if a prosthetic is requested by the family, an intense training program and careful follow-up, may improve the success rate of prosthetic incorporation.

Another investigation evaluated 207 patients with a diagnosis of a congenital transverse deficiency of the forearm and found that a large majority of the patients had nubbins, skin invaginations, or bone abnormalities that suggested a continuum with symbrachydactyly (as a developmental abnormality) rather than an isolated amputation.[32]

POLYDACTYLY-TRIPHALANGEAL THUMB

A recent investigation of 19 patients with more than 7-year follow-up demonstrated the difficulty in treatment of radial polydactyly. While overall function was considered satisfactory in these patients, an objective assessment demonstrated 14 of the 19 thumbs had only fair or poor results.[33] In another study of 106 cases of Wassel type IV thumbs with more than 3-year follow-up, the results were fair or poor when the excised digit was more than 75% of the size of the preserved digit. Additionally, the authors divided the thumbs into subtypes and the two subtypes with cartilaginous interconnections (without bony connection) had a worse outcome.[34]

Two recent articles present outcomes of the Bilhaut-Cloquet procedure. The first report demonstrated excellent aesthetic outcome in a modification of the classic Bilhaut-Cloquet procedure for Wassel type II and III thumbs.[35] Instead of merging the two thumbs centrally (with the risks of nail ridging, physeal closure, and joint asymmetry), the majority of one thumb is enhanced with the lateral pulp of the other. Motion is preserved, the nail appearance is good, and growth arrest was not seen. The second article detailed the use of the procedure for types III, IV, and VII thumbs.[36] The authors reported good results with a normal-sized thumb and good function. The authors preserved a single nail when the nail width was greater than 70% of the opposite side; otherwise the nails were merged as classically described.

Additionally, there were two outcome articles on triphalangeal thumbs.[37,38] One reported good results for both function and aesthetics with a two-stage procedure. In the first stage, the proximal interphalangeal joint joint is excised and the metacarpal had corrective osteotomy. In the second stage, an opposition transfer is performed. The other investigation grouped patients by subtypes and recommended early (1–2 years of age) excision of the accessory phalanx and collateral ligament repair or partial epiphysis resection (rather than osteotomy).

NONVASCULARIZED AND VASCULARIZED TOE TRANSFERS

Recent reports do little to clarify the controversial role of nonvascularized toe phalanx transfers. One recent investigation, in which most transfers were performed between the ages of 1 and 2 years, demonstrated that only 4 of 18 phalanges maintained an open physis and that growth gains at 7 years were modest (75% of contralateral toe phalanx).[39] In another investigation, 64 of 113 nonvascularized free phalanx transfers demonstrated growth with another 22 demonstrating resorption (which increased with patient age).[40] However, the authors of the second article were optimistic about the technique and recommended early surgery for greater growth potential. The practical use of the technique remains questionable and, when used, these data of equivocal outcomes are helpful for preoperative counseling.

A report of 14 double-vascularized toe transfers found that all toes were mobile and sensate with improved function and appearance of the upper extremity. However, all hands needed secondary surgical procedures.[41] The psychological aspects of toe to hand transfer were evaluated in 32 congenital cases. The results were overall quite positive in respect to aesthetic and functional satisfaction with surgery.[42]

DIGITAL CALLOTASIS

Four articles reported the outcome of callotasis for congenitally short digits, most commonly in symbrachydactyly.[43–46] All four reported successful lengthening of metacarpals and phalanges although complications were common. When the studies are taken together, the fixator remained in place (distraction plus consolidation) for approximately 85 days, the length gains ranged from

11 to 24 mm, and the percentage length gain ranged from 44% to 82%. The use of an intramedullary Kirschner wire to help stabilize the bone during lengthening was recommended in two of the articles. As our understanding of bone growth and healing progresses, these procedures are likely to become more reliable though the use of various growth factors.

SYNDACTYLY

Six articles on syndactyly provide multiple surgical techniques. Three articles describe techniques to avoid skin grafts in cutaneous syndactyly. One describes an "open" technique using multiple flaps and limited closure.[47] Another describes the use of aggressive defatting of the fingers.[48] The third describes the use of a dorsal metacarpal flap.[49] The last technique uses the advanced dorsal skin to recreate the commissural flap and avoid skin grafting; however, opponents of the technique note that it leaves a more prominent dorsal scar. A technique for partial syndactyly reconstruction using the three square flap was also described.[50] The issue of lateral nail fold creation for complete syndactyly was addressed in a report of the outcome in 75 fingertips. The Buck-Gramcko pulp flaps provided a successful technique that allowed avoidance of grafting.[51] Finally, Friedman and Wood[52] reviewed the use of the dorsal transposition flap for first web space reconstruction; satisfactory results were reported.

APERT'S SYNDROME

Three articles on Apert's Syndrome provide guidance for the reconstruction. Chang and colleagues[53] reported on 10 patients treated with early bilateral border digit separation and subsequent unilateral central syndactyly reconstruction. Most of the syndactylies were complex and the thumb frequently had corrective osteotomy (11 thumbs). Low revision rates with good functional outcomes and high parental satisfaction are reported. Fearon[54] reported early treatment (syndactyly release) and late treatment (functional osteotomies). Most patients required a two-stage operation to provide 10 fingers with no ray amputations performed. Low revision rates and high satisfaction were reported. Van Heest and colleagues[55] reported a treatment protocol based on classification; either a three- or four-fingered hand was created with a two-stage operation.

OTHER CONGENITAL ANOMALIES

Two articles report treatment of macrodactyly. The first describes a two-stage debulking and phalangectomy (for shortening) that produced a good aesthetic outcome in 12 of 23 children with macrodactyly.[56] Only two required amputation. In another report of 23 patients, 65% had more than two operations; length was closely restored to normal but the fingers had a greater circumference (approximately 120%) of the opposite side and also had decreased motion.[57] The authors concluded that epiphysiodesis was successful, but hypertrophic nerve resection was not. Macrodactyly remains largely unexplained, and bench research on differential growth offers the hope of information and more appropriate molecular-based therapy.

Rider and colleagues[58] reported on the Snow-Littler procedure for central deficiency in 12 hands. Good results were reported with no major flap necrosis; derotational osteotomies were required in three transposed index fingers in patients with transverse metacarpal ligament reconstruction.

Smith and Grobbelaar[59] reported on 18 fingers with camptodactyly. Good results with a complete release of all involved structures were demonstrated; the authors recommend against surgery for patients with less than a 60° contracture because these patients were considered to have minimal functional problems. Foucher and colleagues[60] provided a useful treatment algorithm for camptodactyly based on clinical examination and the function of the involved anatomic structures.

Finally, clinodactyly is often caused by an abnormally-shaped middle phalanx in the small finger. Cauoette-Laberge and colleagues[61] reported a simple physiolysis with fat interposition with good correction. Patients treated before 6 years of age and those with a trapezoidal middle phalanx had the best correction.

SUMMARY

The last 12 years has seen steady progress in our understanding and treatment of congenital hand anomalies. The multiple articles that have added to our core knowledge have been included in this review. The future of progress in the treatment of congenital hand anomalies is bright, and the areas of tissue engineering and gene therapy offer the most hope for dramatic treatment progress.

REFERENCES

1. Isogai N, Landis W, Kim TH, et al. Formation of phalanges and small joints by tissue-engineering. J Bone Joint Surg Am 1999;81(3):306–16.
2. Naruse T, Takahara M, Takagi M, et al. Early morphological changes leading to central polydactyly,

syndactyly, and central deficiencies: an experimental study in rats. J Hand Surg [Am] 2007;32(9):1413–7.

3. Evans CH, Rosier RN. Molecular biology in orthopaedics: the advent of molecular orthopaedics. J Bone Joint Surg Am 2005;87(11):2550–64.

4. James MA, Green HD, McCarroll HR Jr, et al. The association of radial deficiency with thumb hypoplasia. J Bone Joint Surg Am 2004;86(10):2196–205.

5. James MA, McCarroll HR Jr, Manske PR. The spectrum of radial longitudinal deficiency: a modified classification. J Hand Surg [Am] 1999;24(6):1145–55.

6. Tytherleigh-Strong G, Hooper G. The classification of phocomelia. J Hand Surg [Br] 2003;28(3):215–7.

7. Goldfarb CA, Manske PR, Busa R, et al. Upper-extremity phocomelia reexamined: a longitudinal dysplasia. J Bone Joint Surg Am 2005;87(12):2639–48.

8. Goldfarb CA, Klepps SJ, Dailey LA, et al. Functional outcome after centralization for radius dysplasia. J Hand Surg [Am] 2002;27(1):118–24.

9. Geck MJ, Dorey F, Lawrence JF, et al. Congenital radius deficiency: radiographic outcome and survivorship analysis. J Hand Surg [Am] 1999;24(6):1132–44.

10. Damore E, Kozin SH, Thoder JJ, et al. The recurrence of deformity after surgical centralization for radial clubhand. J Hand Surg [Am] 2000;25(4):745–51.

11. Lamb DW, Scott H, Lam WL, et al. Operative correction of radial club hand: a long-term follow-up of centralization of the hand on the ulna. The Journal of Hand Surgery: Journal of the British Society for Surgery of the Hand 1997;22(4):533–6.

12. Sestero AM, Van Heest A, Agel J. Ulnar growth patterns in radial longitudinal deficiency. J Hand Surg [Am] 2006;31(6):960–7.

13. Vilkki SK. Distraction and microvascular epiphysis transfer for radial club hand. J Hand Surg [Br] 1998;23(4):445–52.

14. Taghinia AH, Al-Sheikh AA, Upton J. Preoperative soft-tissue distraction for radial longitudinal deficiency: an analysis of indications and outcomes. Plast Reconstr Surg 2007;120(5):1305–12 [discussion: 1313–04].

15. Sabharwal S, Finuoli AL, Ghobadi F. Pre-centralization soft tissue distraction for Bayne type IV congenital radial deficiency in children. J Pediatr Orthop 2005;25(3):377–81.

16. Goldfarb CA, Murtha YM, Gordon JE, et al. Soft-tissue distraction with a ring external fixator before centralization for radial longitudinal deficiency. J Hand Surg [Am] 2006;31(6):952–9.

17. Matsuno T, Ishida O, Sunagawa T, et al. Radius lengthening for the treatment of Bayne and Klug type II and type III radial longitudinal deficiency. J Hand Surg [Am] 2006;31(5):822–9.

18. Mo JH, Manske PR. Surgical treatment of type 0 radial longitudinal deficiency. J Hand Surg [Am] 2004;29(6):1002–9.

19. Pickford MA, Scheker LR. Distraction lengthening of the ulna in radial club hand using the Ilizarov technique. J Hand Surg [Br] 1998;23(2):186–91.

20. Peterson BM, McCarroll HR Jr, James MA. Distraction lengthening of the ulna in children with radial longitudinal deficiency. J Hand Surg [Am] 2007;32(9):1402–7.

21. Horii E, Nakamura R, Nakao E, et al. Distraction lengthening of the forearm for congenital and developmental problems. J Hand Surg [Br] 2000;25(1):15–21.

22. Goldfarb CA, Wall L, Manske PR. Radial longitudinal deficiency: the incidence of associated medical and musculoskeletal conditions. J Hand Surg [Am] 2006;31(7):1176–82.

23. Clark DI, Chell J, Davis TR. Pollicisation of the index finger. A 27-year follow-up study. J Bone Joint Surg Br 1998;80(4):631–5.

24. Graham TJ, Louis DS. A comprehensive approach to surgical management of the type IIIA hypoplastic thumb. J Hand Surg [Am] 1998;23(1):3–13.

25. Shibata M, Yoshizu T, Seki T, et al. Reconstruction of a congenital hypoplastic thumb with use of a free vascularized metatarsophalangeal joint. J Bone Joint Surg Am 1998;80(10):1469–76.

26. Goldfarb CA, Deardorff V, Chia B, et al. Objective features and aesthetic outcome of pollicized digits compared with normal thumbs. J Hand Surg [Am] 2007;32(7):1031–6.

27. Cole RJ, Manske PR. Classification of ulnar deficiency according to the thumb and first web. J Hand Surg [Am] 1997;22(3):479–88.

28. Havenhill TG, Manske PR, Patel A, et al. Type 0 ulnar longitudinal deficiency. J Hand Surg [Am] 2005;30(6):1288–93.

29. Elhassan BT, Biafora S, Light T. Clinical manifestations of type IV ulna longitudinal dysplasia. J Hand Surg [Am] 2007;32(7):1024–30.

30. James MA, Bagley AM, Brasington K, et al. Impact of prostheses on function and quality of life for children with unilateral congenital below-the-elbow deficiency. J Bone Joint Surg Am 2006;88(11):2356–65.

31. Davids JR, Wagner LV, Meyer LC, et al. Prosthetic management of children with unilateral congenital below-elbow deficiency. J Bone Joint Surg Am 2006;88(6):1294–300.

32. Kallemeier PM, Manske PR, Davis B, et al. An assessment of the relationship between congenital transverse deficiency of the forearm and symbrachydactyly. J Hand Surg [Am] 2007;32(9):1408–12.

33. Larsen M, Nicolai JP. Long-term follow-up of surgical treatment for thumb duplication. J Hand Surg [Br] 2005;30(3):276–81.

34. Horii E, Nakamura R, Sakuma M, et al. Duplicated thumb bifurcation at the metacarpophalangeal joint

level: factors affecting surgical outcome. J Hand Surg [Am] 1997;22(4):671–9.

35. Baek GH, Gong HS, Chung MS, et al. Modified Bilhaut-Cloquet procedure for Wassel type-II and III polydactyly of the thumb. J Bone Joint Surg Am 2007;89(3):534–41.

36. Tonkin MA, Bulstrode NW. The Bilhaut-Cloquet procedure for Wassel types III, IV and VII thumb duplication. J Hand Surg Eur Vol 2007;32(6):684–93.

37. El-Karef E. The non-opposable triphalangeal thumb: a new technique of management. J Hand Surg [Br] 2004;29(6):544–51.

38. Horii E, Nakamura R, Makino H. Triphalangeal thumb without associated abnormalities: clinical characteristics and surgical outcomes. Plast Reconstr Surg 2001;108(4):902–7.

39. Tonkin MA, Deva AK, Filan SL. Long term follow-up of composite non-vascularized toe phalanx transfers for aphalangia. J Hand Surg [Br] 2005;30(5):452–8.

40. Gohla T, Metz C, Lanz U. Non-vascularized free toe phalanx transplantation in the treatment of symbrachydactyly and constriction ring syndrome. J Hand Surg [Br] 2005;30(5):446–51.

41. Holder CVAN, Giele H, Gilbert A. Double second toe transfer in congenital hand anomalies. The Journal of Hand Surgery: Journal of the British Society for Surgery of the Hand 1999;24(4):471–5.

42. Bellew M, Kay SP. Psychological aspects of toe to hand transfer in children. Comparison of views of children and their parents. J Hand Surg [Br] 1999;24(6):712–8.

43. Dhalla R, Strecker W, Manske PR. A comparison of two techniques for digital distraction lengthening in skeletally immature patients. J Hand Surg [Am] 2001;26(4):603–10.

44. Miyawaki T, Masuzawa G, Hirakawa M, et al. Bone-lengthening for symbrachydactyly of the hand with the technique of callus distraction. J Bone Joint Surg Am 2002;84(6):986–91.

45. Kato H, Minami A, Suenaga N, et al. Callotasis lengthening in patients with brachymetacarpia. J Pediatr Orthop 2002;22(4):497–500.

46. Pensler JM, Carroll NC, Cheng LF. Distraction osteogenesis in the hand. Plast Reconstr Surg 1998;102(1):92–5.

47. Withey SJ, Kangesu T, Carver N, et al. The open finger technique for the release of syndactyly. J Hand Surg [Br] 2001;26(1):4–7.

48. Greuse M, Coessens BC. Congenital syndactyly: defatting facilitates closure without skin graft. J Hand Surg [Am] 2001;26(4):589–94.

49. Sherif MM. V-Y dorsal metacarpal flap: a new technique for the correction of syndactyly without skin graft. Plast Reconstr Surg 1998;101(7):1861–6.

50. Bandoh Y, Yanai A, Seno H. The three-square-flap method for reconstruction of minor syndactyly. J Hand Surg [Am] 1997;22(4):680–4.

51. Golash A, Watson JS. Nail fold creation in complete syndactyly using Buck-Gramcko pulp flaps. J Hand Surg [Br] 2000;25(1):11–4.

52. Friedman R, Wood VE. The dorsal transposition flap for congenital contractures of the first web space: a 20-year experience. J Hand Surg [Am] 1997;22(4):664–70.

53. Chang J, Danton TK, Ladd AL, et al. Reconstruction of the hand in Apert syndrome: a simplified approach. Plast Reconstr Surg 2002;109(2):465–70 [discussion: 471].

54. Fearon JA. Treatment of the hands and feet in Apert syndrome: an evolution in management. Plast Reconstr Surg 2003;112(1):1–12 [discussion: 13–19].

55. Van Heest AE, House JH, Reckling WC. Two-stage reconstruction of apert acrosyndactyly. J Hand Surg [Am] 1997;22(2):315–22.

56. Kotwal PP, Farooque M. Macrodactyly. J Bone Joint Surg Br 1998;80(4):651–3.

57. Ishida O, Ikuta Y. Long-term results of surgical treatment for macrodactyly of the hand. Plast Reconstr Surg 1998;102(5):1586–90.

58. Rider MA, Grindel SI, Tonkin MA, et al. An experience of the Snow-Littler procedure. J Hand Surg [Br] 2000;25(4):376–81.

59. Smith PJ, Grobbelaar AO. Camptodactyly: a unifying theory and approach to surgical treatment. J Hand Surg [Am] 1998;23(1):14–9.

60. Foucher G, Lorea P, Khouri RK, et al. Camptodactyly as a spectrum of congenital deficiencies: a treatment algorithm based on clinical examination. Plast Reconstr Surg 2006;117(6):1897–905.

61. Caouette-Laberge L, Laberge C, Egerszegi EP, et al. Physiolysis for correction of clinodactyly in children. J Hand Surg [Am] 2002;27(4):659–65.

Index

Note: Page numbers of article titles are in **boldface** type.

Hand Clin 25 (2009) 301–304
doi:10.1016/S0749-0712(09)00015-8

hand.theclinics.com

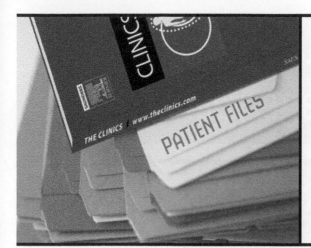
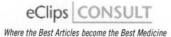
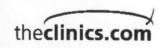

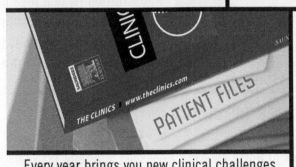

Moving?

Make sure your subscription moves with you!

To notify us of your new address, find your **Clinics Account Number** (located on your mailing label above your name), and contact customer service at:

E-mail: elspcs@elsevier.com

800-654-2452 (subscribers in the U.S. & Canada)
314-453-7041 (subscribers outside of the U.S. & Canada)

Fax number: 314-523-5170

Elsevier Periodicals Customer Service
11830 Westline Industrial Drive
St. Louis, MO 63146

*To ensure uninterrupted delivery of your subscription, please notify us at least 4 weeks in advance of move.

ELSEVIER

Printed and bound by CPI Group (UK) Ltd, Croydon, CR0 4YY

03/10/2024

01040354-0014